First Steps to Fitness

The step-by-step guide for complete beginners

Ann Goodsell

BLOOMSBURY

The publishers would like to thank:
Photography: Paul Lawrence
Hair and make-up: Red Welsh
Technical adviser: Lennie Botter
Leotards: The King's Road Sporting Club

The information in this book was correct to the best of the editor's and publisher's belief at the time of going
to press. While no responsibility can be accepted for errors or omissions, the editor and publisher would
welcome corrections and suggestions for material to include in subsequent editions of this book.

This edition first published in 1996 by
Bloomsbury Publishing plc
2 Soho Square
London, W1V 6HB

A copy of the CIP entry for this book is available from the British Library

ISBN 0 7475 2254 5

Cover design by Slatter Anderson
Designed by Planet X and Purple & Sabre
Printed and bound in Great Britain by Jarrold & Sons Ltd

CONTENTS

Author's acknowledgments
I would like to say a big thank you to my husband, family and friends for supporting me through this challenging time. Thanks also to my editor, to all the caring people in the health and fitness business and especially to Lennie Botter for her invaluable help and support during the making of this book.

First Steps to Fitness is not about a two-week makeover, nor is it intended for people who already have a fitness regime that they have no trouble sticking to. It is for those who do nothing and have realized that as time ticks away, their bodies will enable them to do even less than they can today. It is also for life – it's about gradually changing those habits that chip away at confidence, self-esteem and ability to deal with life's ups and downs.

You've taken the first step by buying this book, so you've acknowledged that you need to make some changes in your life. You've realized that this is not a dress rehearsal – this is the only life you are going to get and it makes sense to live it as long as you can, in the best possible health.

Life often seems like a game of snakes and ladders, one day you are four rungs up the ladder, feeling good, relationship fine, children OK, bills not too piled up – you're in control. Then, something happens, and one (often minor) event – the car won't start, the freezer packs up – sets you sliding out of control down a snake until you wonder if you are ever going to start climbing again. If that scenario sounds familiar, this book is for you.

This is about being kind to yourself, gently and slowly. It's about setting yourself realistic goals that are easy to achieve, so that you will not be disappointed. It's about changing lifelong habits gradually – yes, they can be broken, no matter how firmly entrenched you think they are. And it's about getting your body moving, through aerobic activity (walking) and exercise (to build some strength).

Food and fitness go together

Along with exercise in your daily life, you need to eat well. Starving your body does not make you lose weight and can do long-term damage. Quick weight loss prevents the absorption of essential vitamins and minerals, causes headaches and violent mood swings, and upsets the body's hormones. Stop worrying about your weight, stop dieting, and start doing something positive instead.

If you eat well, you will have more energy to exercise, be more motivated to try something new and feel better able to cope when the pressure is on. This can only improve the quality of your life.

But I don't like exercise, I hear you say. Perhaps you simply haven't found a way of getting some exercise that suits you yet. One step at a time, one poor eating habit at a time, and you will start to see positive results and look and feel better. That, in itself, should be enough to spur you on further. You may not lose 10 kg, but you may lose 5 kg over the 12 weeks that this course is designed to take. And this is just the beginning. This book is going to ease you into fitness and good eating habits and help you appreciate that food is not your enemy, but your fuel, as essential to your wellbeing as petrol is to the car.

When you eat good foods and get some regular exercise into your life, you function more efficiently and your blood sugar levels stay even, which helps to prevent violent mood swings and stops you reaching for the biscuit tin for a few minutes' comfort. Now is the time to start gradually changing and adapting your lifestyle to make a healthier, more relaxed you.

Think about when you last felt comfortable with how you looked and felt, and when you last enjoyed the life you are living. If it was more than a year ago, think long and hard about what has happened to make you out of control of your exercise and eating habits and leave you no time for yourself?

Now think about how long it is going to take you to put some of it right. Realistically, probably a couple of years, depending on how many habits you need to break and how hard you are prepared to work at it. Start slowly with one or two things a week so that you don't find it too stressful. Forget the word diet and all the bad feelings that are associated with it, and start eating more unrefined foods to give you energy.

FIRST STEPS TO FITNESS

Q Can I look like a B?

A We can all aspire toward B since we can all use more muscle and less fat. If you lean toward A and lack muscle tone, you can use heavier weights and low repetitions to build muscle while eating more carbohydrates and protein. If you are closer to C, you can lose body fat through aerobic work, and gradually cutting down on fats and upping your intake of carbohydrate.

Q I'm a combination of all three body types. What should I do?

A Aerobic work will reduce body fat, and using weights will strengthen your body.

Q Where do I start?

A Like everybody else, you need to start building a basic fitness level. You need to increase your aerobic capacity gradually over the 12 weeks, at the same time as you gain some strength in all the major muscle groups. Master the technique for these important exercises, do them well, and work toward your goals. Enjoy these 12 weeks, they are the beginnings of a new you. Go for it!

Standing tall: your posture

Look around you at the way people stand and how they sit – necks craned, backs curved, sagging tummies. Now try to catch yourself in a shop window or mirror. Could you do with some posture checking? Sitting at a PC all day, or spending a long time driving can have a devastating effect on your body over months and years, especially if all you do when you get home is slump in front of the TV week in week out.

The real problem with poor posture is that strain in one area sets off a chain reaction in another. If your back aches, another part of your body (usually the next weakest) works harder to compensate and before you know it, you've got pain somewhere else, and so on. Prevention is better than a cure, so straighten up, think tall and walk tall and work toward keeping your body tall and proud.

How? Well, you start by putting a little strength into your muscles, not body building but body toning. Toned muscles support the skeleton, keeping it upright and enabling you to do just about everything, from playing football to washing the dishes. If you do not start to tone your body now, the natural degeneration we all experience as we age will be far greater.

You may well suffer from the breakdown of cartilage around the knee, shoulder, hip and elbow joints and depletion of cushioning between the joints. This can cause severe pain which in turn makes you move and sit in ways that you are unaccustomed to, in order to ease the pain. And there you have that chain reaction again.

Exercises to support and strengthen the torso such as lower abdominal raises (p. 52) keep your pelvis (your centre of movement), working smoothly. Lower back raises (p. 146) support and strengthen the complex network of muscles of the lower back.

Posture and workouts

Right from week 1, it is important to work on improving your posture. Poor posture will make your workout less effective and, more importantly, it could lead to injury. Start by doing the exercises slowly so that you are totally in control of your movements. By the end of the 12 weeks, you will be standing taller, feeling and looking slimmer, and will feel stronger in your back and abdomen.

There are two types of posture, that of rest and that of movement. At rest, stand or sit tall, with relaxed shoulders and chest; lift your ribcage and, as you do so, you will automatically feel your back straighten up. Pull your abdomen in – this may feel strange at first, but it will gradually become automatic. If you are standing at rest, tilt your hip area (pelvis) forward slightly (it is only slight).

Poor posture is very obvious when you move. Bad body alignment through the foot, up the shins and into the knee area, up the back of the legs into the pelvis and lower back, up the back, and into the shoulders and the neck is caused by not placing the foot down properly. Put your heel down first, then roll the rest of your foot down to your toes.

- *Poor posture causes aches and pains, which can lead to injuries.*
- *Exercise and good posture make you look good and feel great.*

What is fitness?

Fitness means different things to different people, but it is not simply about how far you can run, how many step classes you do a week or how often you play football or squash. True fitness is about finding a balance in each area of your life, having peace of mind, and leading an active life with a body that can stand the pace. Think about the following areas of your life.

Lifestyle
- Are you happy with your work? Are you in the right job? Do you need a change?
- What is the balance between your work and your personal life? Might it need adjustment?
- Do you find some pleasure in each day? Do you have any hobbies you really enjoy? Do you do any evening classes? How much time do you have to think only about yourself? How many minutes do you have to exercise your body?

Emotions
- Are you generally happy? Sad? OK? What makes you any of these?
- Do you feel in control or are you always trying to catch up with something?
- Are you nervous? Are you sensitive to what others think and say?
- Do you suffer from depression? Are you anxious? Do you feel generally stable?
- Do you feel alive?
- Does food control you? How much do you think about it?

Socially
- What is your relationship like with your partner? Family? Friends? Colleagues?
- Are you an introvert, keeping everything to yourself? Or an extrovert, generally open about most things?

- Do you have any personal space? Sometimes? Often? Never?
- Can you communicate with people?
- Is eating out or eating in a problem for you?

Spiritually
- Are you comfortable about yourself? Do you feel content?
- Do your values give you good feelings?
- Do you have a moral sense that is real for you?
- Can you do anything you put your mind to?

In your brain
- Do you have a good level of concentration?
- How is your memory? Good? Poor? As good as anybody else's?
- Do you say yes when you mean no?
- Can you make a decision?
- Do you know that what you eat affects your mental ability?

Activity
- Do you move your body – walking, jogging, racket sport, swimming, exercise class? Do you do anything that makes you move over and above your usual daily activity?
- When was the last time you took a good deep breath and filled your lungs with oxygen?
- Can you feel – really feel – a muscle anywhere in your body?
- Are you able to do what you want: Reach to a shelf? Tie a shoelace? Do up a back zip? Pick up the kids' toys?

What do you want?

Be honest with yourself about what you want from life and what you need. Start today to think about exactly what you do aspire to.

Setting your goals

It is important to start with realistic challenges that you can cope with today. Your goals may alter as you develop and change, but it's always best to start small and take one step at a time.

Have a long bath, add your favourite oils or salts, and really relax and think about yourself. Dry off and take your measurements – chest, waist, hips. Are they a bit of a surprise? Then stand in front of a full-length mirror and take a good look at yourself. Look at all your curves and contours, really study your shape. Do you like what you see? Are you in proportion? Which is your predominant body type (pp 6–7)?

Look at your shoulders. Are they square, rounded, sloping, large or small?

An easy way to improve the appearance of your shoulders is to alternate the shoulder or arm on which you carry a bag. Try a rucksack, which distributes the weight of what you are carrying across both shoulders equally. (This might feel strange at first, but if you give it time, your body will realign itself.)

If you sit at a desk all day, check the position of your seat, and if you use a VDU check your position in relation to the screen. Your feet should be flat on the floor and you should not have to hunch your shoulders to use the keyboard properly, nor look down or up to see the display. If you have problems with this, talk to your employer. From 1996, employers will be legally bound to ensure that office furniture falls within government guidelines – so make a fuss now.

If you drive a lot, check your seat position too. Driving automatically tends to make people tense; sitting badly simply compounds the problem.

From week five there is an exercise especially for the shoulders, which also helps take pressure off your back.

What kind of a chest do you have? Is it large, small, high, low, flabby?

Male or female, you can improve the look of your chest and the tone of your muscles there. Female breasts are not muscle, but fat and ligament, but working on your chest will improve the muscles supporting them, giving your breasts better definition. A good chest improves the appearance of the male body enormously.

Study your legs. Are they short, long, large, small, big thighs, small thighs? Do they rub together or could you push a bus through them? Are your knees puffy, bony, sticking out, OK?

Knees are very vulnerable and need special attention, so from week two there is an exercise designed to improve this area so that you can walk without risking injury. Improving the look of your legs take time, because they are strong to begin with. Walking and strength training – which comes in week eleven with an exercise for the legs and bottom – will both help, as will a healthier diet, but be prepared for it to take months rather than weeks before you see real improvements in your legs. Remember that you cannot spot reduce fat, but you can spot tone certain areas and your legs will certainly improve in shape if you work them.

Are your calves bulbous, tiny, short, long, good or bad? How do you feel about them?

From week six, you can work on improving the strength and tone of these muscles. If you have small calves, you can certainly give them some definition; if they are large to start with, you are never going to get rid of them, but you can tone them and once you have improved the look of your legs overall, your calves will seem less prominent.

Are your arms like dough, or are they like bits of string on the end of your shoulders? Are they shapely or ugly? What do you think? Can you see any muscle? Do the backs of your arms sway when you move?

The upper body takes to toning very well and you will quickly see results here. The exercises for weeks four and seven are for the backs and fronts of your arms and if you do them well and with correct technique, you should notice improvements within a matter of weeks.

Really study yourself. Be honest. Absorb what you see, take it all in. What are you feeling? What are you thinking? Start writing! These are very personal thoughts and ones that you need to face in order to arrive at goals that you can attain. This is the hardest thing you will have to do. The rest can only go toward improving what you already have. Ask yourself the following questions: What am I looking for? What do I hope to achieve? Why am I doing it? Is it for me or somebody else?

Making it real

Now analyse how realistic your goals are, and understand what they involve in terms of time, effort and discomfort. You must want this badly enough. Write your big goal at the beginning of each week of the diary as a constant reminder.

What do I want? Good strong thighs? A firmer bottom? Do I want to develop the shape of my chest? Strengthen my back? Lower back? Build my arms? Improve my range of movement? Improve my posture? Run 1 km, 5 km, a half marathon? Or do you simply want to feel and look better and to have some of what all those other active people have – a sparkle in their eyes, a skip in their stride, great presence, an endless supply of energy and an abundance of attitude to enjoy life to the full and to live positively.

If you are unhappy with something, change it or at least put it on the list of goals to work toward. Take your time and really think about what exactly you want to achieve. Is it possible? How much time can you honestly put in to reach your goals? Remember that healthy eating and exercise are to become a part of your daily lifestyle – unrealistic goals from the start will take you nowhere. This is about exchanging old habits for new ones, habits that may have been with you since you were a child. Be realistic about what you can do and keep the goals small to start with, until you have broken the vicious circle of trying for too much, failing, and feeling worse than when you started. Everything in life can become easier to deal with as you learn to master yourself.

A stubborn habit (tea, coffee, chocolate) is going to take at least four weeks to break (see p. 23). If you fail, don't pick another goal, stick with this one until you crack it, then move on to the next week. In this way, every time you tackle something new, you have the satisfaction of success behind you – you know you can do it. Some things take one month to master, some six – it really doesn't matter as long as you stick with it.

SMALL GOALS	MEDIUM GOALS	BIG GOALS
Walk 15–30mins daily	Start jogging 3-4 times per week	Complete a 10 km fun run next year
Cut down on fat consumption to lose 500g a week,	To do aerobic activities gradually building up to 3 times per week	To lose 5-10 kg in weight
Play bat and ball with the kids once a week	Play with the kids in the park/ garden regularly twice a week	To be active in the kids' sports day
Start the 12 week walking/ exercise programme	Try circuit training in the local gym/ church hall	Join local sports club
Do a beginners' aerobics class once a week	Do an aerobics class twice a week	Do an aerobics class three times a week
Cut out two fat- and sugar-laden foods	Do aerobic work 3–4 times a to burn and reduce body fat	Get into a suit last worn two years ago
Start swimming a couple of times a week.	Take diving lessons	Learn sub-aqua/ diving
Check out local schools, colleges, for evening classes	Enrol for classes	Try a new hobby

How do you feel today?

Our thoughts and moods affect us from the moment we wake. Even if you wake feeling fine, you can be distressed, angry and frustrated by the time you leave the house. Then you have to get to work and take the children to school – both of which can be stressful, especially if you live in a city. And that is just the start. Throughout the day, moods can change in an instant – only you can control how you feel and how you react to people and events.

Part of the 12-week programme is assessing your moods to see if you are generally a fairly positive person or whether you are normally negative and miserable, and what you want to do about that. Eating good energy-giving foods and taking daily exercise will contribute beyond your wildest dreams to making you feel good, banishing those deep depressions and avoiding those swift mood swings that make you – and everyone around you – feel so bad.

The mood scale will help you to understand your mood swings, not only throughout the day, but from week to week and month to month. Try to fill them in every day, morning and night – you are doing this programme for you and part of it is learning about yourself. Start by thinking about how you felt this morning. Look at the faces and choose the one most appropriate to your feelings when you woke. This has already made you aware of how you are feeling now, so note this down too. The same applies to last thing at night. When you go to bed tonight, look at the faces and see which one fits you best. Are you in a better mood than you were this morning? What has happened to make the day's end so much better or worse than its beginning?

You might find it helps to write a few words to sum up the moment, even if it is something silly. As you work through the 12 weeks, you will be able to see the good and bad days, and so on. The list is endless for all of us – food, exercise, partner, children, family, friends, colleagues. Start to look at what you like, and what you don't like and how you might be able to turn dislikes around. Even if you can't turn every bad mood around, you may find you can do it once, which will give you the heart to try it again. Keep trying: like everything else, the more you practise the better your chances of success.

Use the mood scale to help you assess what kind of workout you had, and how you were affected by your mood. If I go into a session not really wanting to do it, I have to focus hard on what I am doing. As a result I always end up really enjoying it and feel pleased with myself when I have finished. From week 1, you will see and feel a definite difference in your mood before and after exercise. You will experience a feeling of great self-satisfaction, the feeling of accomplishing this for yourself, which in itself is very rewarding. Your body will be revitalized through activity and you will start to feel alive.

As the 12 weeks progress, you will see what exercise has done for you, how it has helped to lift your mood. Have you diverted a bad mood? Have you channelled it into your brisk walking and your exercises? Exercise is a great time to tune out or tune in to something specific, release some of the tension you acquire through life's day-to-day pulse raisers.

Using the mood scale taught me that my mood swings were related to the fact that I was not eating good foods often enough to keep my blood sugar levels even. At the time I was snacking on high-sugar and high-fat foods, coffee and teas, to give me an energy boost, which in fact only cured me for maybe 10–20 minutes, and then I was famished again. Now my body does not go hungry and therefore I now am able to avoid loss of self-control and mood swings.

I travel everywhere with a snack box full of good energy-giving foods and the tantrums have gone. The mood scale has taught me to feel and to think and to know that I am in charge of how I feel.

How hard are you working?

The feeling scale is a simple way to ensure that you are working hard enough to encourage your body to burn food for energy, reduce the amount of body fat you are carrying, and improve your level of all-round fitness. You should not work so hard that you are breathless or unable to hold a conversation. If that happens, ease up so that you are breathing comfortably, but your exercise is still taking a little effort. If you warm up gradually, and resist the temptation to go too fast, you will get through and – equally important – enjoy your exercise session.

If you have been very inactive, your aerobic fitness is going to be poor to start with and you may find that even in the first few days, exercise is hard – somewhere between 15 and 18 on the feeling scale. Don't despair – try walking a bit slower, but for longer. The fitter you become, the easier you will find it to stay between 15 and 18 on the scale for your whole 30-minute walk. The longer you can stay working at this intensity, the more calories you will burn, working toward reducing your body fat and stimulating your metabolic rate still further – all of which leads to improvements in the functioning of your heart and lungs.

If you can afford a pulse monitor and want to learn how to use it, you will get a more accurate picture of exactly how hard you are working. But in the early stages of your route to fitness, the feeling scale is more than enough. You will know when you are working too hard because your body will tell you. Think about how you feel before you start your workout, after your warm-up, during the exercises and directly afterward. Do you think you worked hard enough? Not hard enough? Could you have done a bit more?

Did you enjoy it? Did you find it easy to breathe, or difficult? Were you tired because you had not eaten enough good foods before you started? Over the weeks you will find it increasingly easy to tell how hard you are working as you discover what your threshold is. Remember that the effort and time you spend doing this will be reflected in your overall goals.

The Feeling scale

10 **Very light**   This should be comfortable and not too much effort. This is a good rate at which to start your warm up (see p. 16), during which you should gradually build to a faster pace, getting all your joints moving as you do so.

12 **Light**   You should be breathing slightly heavier now, taking in larger amounts of oxygen to warm all your muscles and prepare them for the workout to come.

15 **Hard**   You are now breathing more heavily and more deeply, and beginning to feel that you are working harder.

16 **Harder**   Although you are breathing more heavily, you

17 **Very hard**   should be able to talk at the same time. Your body should feel as if it is working hard. You are aiming to work at this intensity for as much of your exercise session as you can.

19 **Extra Hard**   You cannot and will not be able to maintain this level of intensity for long. You will feel that you need oxygen and find breathing difficult. You may also feel light-headed and out of control. Slow down gradually: if you stop suddenly, you will feel worse.

20 **Maximum**   Avoid at all costs. You will feel thoroughly breathless, unable to talk and overheated. This is not what it's all about.

Finding time, making the effort

Most sedentary people however are aware that they are not as mobile as they used to be. Some even accept that unexplained aches and pains, problems climbing the stairs and a little breathlessness as they walk to the bus stop are normal. Stop right there!

FIRST STEPS TO FITNESS

Unless you seriously take charge now, what you are feeling will only get much worse as you get older. Ignoring what you feel is reducing your chances of reaching retirement age when you are officially allowed to enjoy the rest of your life.

You get out what you put in, so stop making excuses and get out there!

HOW OFTEN	WHEN IS BEST	I'M TOO BUSY
Every day. Oh no, I hear you cry. It's not that bad, just ease yourself into it one step at a time, starting with a gentle daily walking.	Anytime you can fit it in; I usually work out early in the morning but it may be 9 Or 10pm if I'm working with clients, or slaving over my PC.	Well OK, that's up to you. We all have to find time as best we can. But if you can't find time for yourself, you're not looking after number 1, which isn't doing the rest of the family any good either.
You are the only person who gives an honest answer as to how much exercise you need for maintenance and if you want to go on after the 12 weeks to higher goals.	Try different times of the day. Over the weeks discover when you have most energy. It takes time to make this part of your daily life.	Time is passing quicker than you think. Take stock now and make time for your body.
Once a week is a good start. Pick the hour and work toward making this habitual.	Don't exercise on a full stomach: leave food to digest at least an hour. Keep meals small and light.	If you can't manage the same time every day, mark in the diary when you can fit it in and make it an unbreakable date.
Twice a week of course is better than once but once is better than none. But it's still not quite enough.	Listen to your body. Use the diary to tell you when to exercise, and eat good foods accordingly.	This is a priority in life and if you see it as anything else you are mistaken. Exercise and good eating provide you with the energy to live the life you want and deserve.
Three times a week –now you're talking. This is maintenance, keeping your body at its current level.	Do you get a stitch when you start exercising? You may not be getting enough oxygen in. Lift your ribcage, give your diaphragm a break and allow your lungs to expand fully.	If you have to miss a day then don't get despondent - just look on it as a rest day. Pick up tomorrow where you left off. It's not a problem if you don't let it become one.
Four times per week will see significant changes in your body: you will be sleeping better and feeling more lively during the day. Your legs and buttocks will start to feel firmer, especially if you make each stride and each exercise count. You'll be better able to cope with everyday stress.	If you've got a dog, exercise when you take it out. Like people, dogs need daily exercise to keep fit, healthy and contented.	'Too busy with the children' is not a good enough excuse - take them with you. Go swimming, or walking in the sunshine. They will benefit too. If they are small, use a pool or gym with a crèche; if there isn't one, hassle until there is - OK, yours may be grown, but someone else will benefit.
Five times a week means your are serious about reaching your goals - this is the one that shows your body that you mean business. You will now start to boost your metabolic rate (see p. 00), as long as you are eating good foods.	If you are feeling below par, a hard workout will not shake it off. Listen to your body and take a walk instead.	There is always tomorrow if you miss today for genuine reasons.
The big six will give you a great buzz as you start to see your body shape change. Your ability to keep going improves and you feel proud and full of energy.	Bandaging an injury is not the answer - you may cause damage. Go to see a sports injuries specialist, stop heavy workouts and do lots of stretching.	Get out first thing in the morning while the rest of the world is asleep. This is great in summer when you can watch the sun rise - a real high.
Rest days are important. No-one is invincible, so don't overdo it. If you do, your body does not have any reserve energy, which makes you susceptible to illness. Listen to your body and rest when you need to. Of course your daily walk is a part of your life now – a treat for your body, so respect this.	The less you use your body, the more likely it is that bits will start to deteriorate and its shape will start to go. Start now - give yourself and anyone else you care about a body to be proud of. One that works efficiently and effectively every day.	Friends and mothers-in-law love babysitting so ask yours to. Look for different ways that you can get some time to yourself to exercise, relax and pamper yourself. We all can make excuses for not doing things – sometimes obstacles are genuine, but you can make choices and these choices reflect your goals. Spend some time thinking about ways to fit it all in. You can do it!

We all need support at some time in our lives. Why not do the 12-week plan of action with a friend or your partner? You'll be suprised how good this can make you both feel.

If you can't manage to get out with a friend more than once or twice a week, fine – it makes your personal workouts more of a challenge.

If a friend or partner can find the time with all his or her commitments, then so can you.

Burning calories

Unless you challenge your body to move, and you watch how much you eat and the quality of what you eat, your body will store excess as fat. Every time you stop working toward making your body look and feel good, your metabolic rate slows and you slip back to a state of low – or no – energy, high levels of body fat and a reduced range of movement around your joints. This puts stress on the joints, and as your body starts to slip out of alignment your muscles start to weaken, which can cause injury or even disability. Your body needs you to exercise daily, beyond your normal day-to-day running about, to keep it functioning at a good level.

The metabolic rate – the rate at which we burn calories – slows down without activity. If you do nothing over and above your usual daily activities, as you age the percentage of body fat you carry increases, so your percentage of lean tissue decreases and your aerobic capacity is poor. Before you know it, you're feeling neither good nor happy and are looking around you wondering what has happened to your body.

Dieting does not work. It causes your body to go into starvation mode, forcing it to lose necessary fluids, and eat away at lean muscle tissue in order to lose those first few kilos in weight. When you stop dieting, you replace the fluids but the lean muscle tissue only comes back when you start exercising, and building some strength. What happens instead is that the food you eat is stored as fat. The more you yo-yo diet, the more fat cells in the body will multiply. The only way to shift unwanted fat is to walk, exercise your heart, exercise your body, breathe, eat good foods, and burn up calories as fuel. Stop worrying about the scales and start working your body.

Start with small daily activities that involve a bit of a challenge, such as taking the stairs at work or walking up the escalator at the station, walk to the next bus stop, play with the children – really play, as in running with them rather than standing around watching – stop using the remote control for everything (consider how much energy you use pressing the button compared to physically moving from one side of the room to the other), wash the car yourself (this is easier if you invest in some quality shampoo) ... the list is endless. If you consider any of these things hard work now, just stop and think how difficult they are going to be in 10 years' time, or 20.

The point here is that you burn far more calories washing your own car than you do by sitting in it while a machine does it for you. But I never stop running round, I hear you say. Unfortunately, your body has adjusted to what you are doing now; it knows exactly how many calories it needs to burn to get you through your hectic daily activities, and it will burn this amount exactly and store the rest. Look at what you do on a day-to-day basis – write it all down, from putting the kettle on to watering the garden – and decide what you can do to increase your level of calorie-burning activities. And it's not simply about burning calories, although that is vital, but it's also about the good feeling that comes from doing something for yourself, however small.

After a few weeks, when your body has slowly adjusted to the extra demands you make on it, stop and remember how uncomfortable the challenge was on the first day. This will help to keep you on the right track, because you do not want to go back to that feeling of finding everything uncomfortable, do you? As you become fitter, your heart and lungs function better. You will also see other benefits. Your body starts to accept that you are not going to starve it, and that you are eating enough for your increased level of daily activities, and gradually raises your metabolic rate. This means that it starts to use the food that you are providing it with more efficiently and effectively, and burns it more quickly. It also starts to burn fat from the stores.

Start slowly, stick with it for the 12.weeks and I guarantee you will stand taller, your body will be firmer, and you will walk with a skip in your stride. You may not have lost 5 kg yet, but you will have had more fun than watching the clock for your next slimming shake.

Calorie-burning activities to start

- Take the stairs at the station.
- If the children go to school locally, leave earlier, and walk them to school.
- At work, take the stairs instead of the lift. If this involves a lot of floors, take it one floor at a time.
- If you have a bicycle, buy a helmet and start pedalling. Most cities have good cycle lanes to make life easier.
- Have you got skates or roller blades (or can you 'borrow' the children's)? These are a great mode of transport, easy and good fun, but make sure you are padded out well.
- Local shops up the road? Leave the car behind and walk.
- Have you booked your holiday? Why not try a cycling holiday? Or a water sports resort?
- What can you add?

Warming up and cooling down

Warming up is one of those things most people know they should be doing, but can't quite be bothered with. Whatever your thoughts on the matter, ban them now: warming up is important.

Your body is made up of a mass of muscles, tendons and ligaments, which connect the body together. In order for you to move at all, they must work together. Imagine you've got an elastic band in your hands. Start pulling it about in different directions, bending it and stretching it. You can feel that it will only stretch so far, and then it will tear or snap. Now take some Plasticine and work it between your fingers, kneading it and bending it. After a couple of minutes gradually make the movements bigger, then try and stretch it to its fullest extent. This time you will find it more pliable, and more willing to stretch further without tearing or breaking. Your muscles work in very much the same way as that elastic band.

If you warm up gradually, starting with small movements and slowly making them bigger, your blood and muscle temperature rises, your joints become lubricated and your synovial fluids (which cushion bones, preventing them rubbing against one another – ouch!) start to work. The muscles become more pliable, and more accommodating, ready to stretch. Only after a warm-up will your body be prepared for the exercise workload to follow, and less likely to be injured in the process.

What to do

Set out on your brisk walk slowly, getting all your joints moving. Start with alternate toe presses – lift up on to the ball of one foot, and slowly roll back down to your heel. Add some ankle circling, small knee lifts. Then move on to small strides, add some shoulder rolls and chest presses, side reaches, neck turns (not backward, which is not good for the spinal cord or vertebrae of the neck), gradually extending your stride and increasing the pace.

Mobilize all your joints, including your wrists and fingers. To be sure to stretch all major muscle groups, either start from your head and work down systematically or work from your feet upward – you will soon develop your own routine. Walking does not just involve the legs, think about the rest of the body and how your walking is affected by it. Check your posture – keep upright. Pump your arms from the shoulder. Remember that if you go too fast too soon, your body will be desperate for extra oxygen, which is uncomfortable and can be dangerous as it increases the blood pressure. If you gradually increase both your body's intake of oxygen and the intensity of your workout, your body will be able to cope with the demands you make of it.

Cooling down is as important as warming up. When you cool down, you lower your body's temperature, and reduce the rate at which the heart pumps blood to your working muscles. At the end of your cool down, you should feel as you did before your warm up, with your heart beating at near-resting rate. If you don't cool down sufficiently, the chances are that blood will pool in your lower limbs and lactic acid will build up. You may feel light headed and your muscles will feel heavy and stiff. You can cool down very easily by gradually reducing the intensity of your brisk walking down to a normal walk, then a very leisurely walk, so that your body returns to normal.

Stretching

So you've done your exercises and your brisk walk, and are feeling good. Now is the time to show your body how much you really appreciate what it has done for you. Make sure that you are warm and have enough layers on to keep your muscles warm and pliable, even though your body has cooled right down. To allow you to exercise, your muscles expand and contract, each time shortening their natural range of movement. This is not a dramatic shortening, but over time, their range of movement is reduced. To keep your body mobile you need to stretch. Over the 12 weeks you will learn one new stretch to complement each week's new exercise. These stretches are easy to do and you should take your time to learn them and to enjoy them.

Ease very gently into all stretches; if it feels uncomfortable, ease back and read the instructions again. If it continues to be uncomfortable, stop and consult your GP, physiotherapist or a qualified gym instructor. Never 'bounce' to take a stretch further. If you bounce into a stretch, the muscle finds it

extremely difficult to relax: basically it fears you are going to bounce too far and cause a strain, tear or worse. For safety's sake, keep your stretches under control.

Taking time out to maintain and improve upon your body's natural abilities and its natural range of movement, is the best form of therapy you can give yourself. Enjoy this time. Remember that quality of movement is quality of life – take that away and what have you got?

What to wear

You don't need the latest fashions in sportswear to do the daily walking and exercises in this book. But it is important to wear something comfortable and loose while you are exercising. Fabrics should allow your body to breathe. Once you decide to up the pace of your fitness programme, by going to classes or to the gym for example, buy the best you can afford: these items are going to be washed over and over again.

Good shoes, however, are a must. Training shoes are designed to absorb the impact of your weight on the ground. They are not cheap, but to work in unsuitable shoes invites injury, so buy the best shoes you can afford. Shop at the end of the day when your feet have expanded. Try some of the movements you do when exercising. Don't expect new shoes to feel as comfortable as your old ones, and remember that if they are too soft to begin with they will not keep their shape. If you are unsure, ask an assistant for advice; say what you are going to be doing in them and how much you can afford. If you don't get the help you need, go somewhere else.

● Always have an extra sweatshirt or teeshirt on hand, especially as you near the end of your cool down. This is the time when the body recovers from the workout, when your muscles can be stretched and returned to their normal range of movement.

- For women a comfortable, supporting sports bra is a must.
- If you decide to swim regularly as part of your exercise plan, buy good-quality swimwear – the chlorine in pools rotsthe fibres and fades the colours of fashion swimwear. You may also need nose and ear plugs, and a hat cuts down drag (and also helps prevent the pool's filters becoming blocked).

What to eat and why

Food is a pure pleasure, there to be enjoyed. You also need it to survive. Eating should be about indulging in good foods that give you plenty of energy. I love food but there came a time when I had to question and look at the content of the food I was eating to become leaner, fitter and full of energy for life.

Certain foods, eaten too regularly, will cause you to carry unnecessary body fat; this builds up over the years and in turn makes you feel sluggish and low in energy. If you want to feel better, you need to make gradual daily changes in what you eat and what you do.

Your body needs good energy-giving foods to work efficiently and effectively, and keep it moving and strong. It does not need the fat- and sugar-laden foods you may have become addicted to (see p. 23). High-fat and high-sugar foods are detrimental to health: they make you fat, affect your energy levels and make you moody. Think of an average day's food intake. How much of what you ate was obviously fat- and sugar-laden? Frightening? But in fact it gets worse. Now that you have remembered all the obvious foods, think a bit harder about all the foods you eat that have hidden fats and sugars. This is almost certainly where you are eating well in excess of the calories you need for the day. And these are the calories that are going to appear exactly where you don't want them – in those areas that already have more than their fair covering of fat.

Are you having difficulties coping daily?	YES ☐ NO ☐
Is your sleep pattern broken regularly?	YES ☐ NO ☐
Are you irritable and stressed out daily?	YES ☐ NO ☐
Are you tired and lacking in energy daily?	YES ☐ NO ☐
Do you lack control with certain foods?	YES ☐ NO ☐
Are you always getting over a cold, or do you feel permanently 'under the weather'?	YES ☐ NO ☐

If you answer yes to two or more of the above questions over the 12 weeks, you really need to address your eating habits as well as your daily activity level, rest time, sleep time and the time you have for yourself. Start looking at how food makes you feel, noting everything (and I mean everything) down in the diary.

If you don't eat good foods and don't exercise, you won't feel 100 per cent. You may feel distant and unable to concentrate on a conversation or the job at hand. Once you adjust to more good, energy-giving foods, you will realize that you are mentally more alert and can concentrate better, you feel more lively and more relaxed, you are not so hungry, and you certainly don't crave quick sugar fixes. You will also find that the niggling cough or snivel you have had for months disappears.

I love my food and, although it has taken me years to learn to cook some well (and I'm still learning), eating good, energy-giving foods is not a problem for me. I like experimenting, experiencing different cultures and all those wonderful secret ingredients that I would not have ventured near several years ago. I finally feel confident that I can present a dinner party to please even the most diehard steak eater.

There is a wonderful supply of fresh foods from all over the world available in your local supermarket, along with wonderfully photographed foods with easy-to-follow recipes in cookbooks and on freebie cooking cards. The sooner you start opening up your eyes and tastebuds to good foods, the sooner you will feel and look great. Don't fight food – eat good food and enjoy it.

A day's food

There is an old saying 'Breakfast like a king, lunch like a prince, dinner like a pauper'. I have a hearty breakfast to set me up for the morning's agenda, a good-sized lunch to see me through the afternoon and a smaller, lighter meal in the evening. And on days when I am very active, I snack throughout the day too.

Plan ahead

A little forward planning can save you a lot of time and allow you to think about and do other things.

- Plan your meals in advance, make a list of what you need to buy when you shop and stick to it – you can't eat what you don't buy.
- Don't shop on an empty stomach. If you really don't have time to eat, have a banana and a couple of rice cakes before you go into the supermarket.
- Read all food labels carefully for the fat, sugar, carbohydrate and sodium content (this obviously is less of an issue when you buy fresh produce).
- Try to cook one new recipe a week. You may not like them all, but at the end of the 12 weeks you might have four or five new dishes in your repertoire.
- Cook larger amounts of rice and pasta than you need for a meal, drain and cool. It will keep in the fridge for several days.
- Make larger quantities of soups and stews – these keep for up to a week.
- Cook a whole chicken or turkey and keep it in the fridge to use in salads, sandwiches, with rice or pasta as a main meal, and in soups and stocks.
- Cook several jacket potatoes at a time and store in the fridge. These only take a few minutes to warm through again in the oven or microwave (personally, I also like them cold).
- Cook larger quantities of any main dishes and freeze the rest into individual portions, use over the coming weeks on 'I can't be bothered to cook' nights.
- Stock up on tinned beans – you never know when you might need them. (Yes, most tins do contain salt and some also have added sugar and ideally it's best to cook your own, but until you know which ones you prefer, it's easier to stick to tins – one step at a time.)

You are active during the day, and therefore this is when you need to eat to refuel your body. Eating very little during the day causes your body to adapt to this low intake and conserve as much energy as possible

(remember that if you don't use it, it will be stored). If you eat a large meal in the evening your body will be only too eager to store as much food energy as possible (as fat) rather than burn it off. So, if you want to boost your metabolism and your energy levels, eat smaller, more frequent good food meals during the day. Keep it simple, and treat yourself occasionally with rich foods. The better the quality of your food, the better the quality of your life.

Breakfast does not have to mean first thing in the morning, when a lot of people don't feel like eating – eat breakfast when you are ready. Get up five minutes early, get yourself ready for the day, do whatever else needs doing, then have something to eat so that you don't stop at the patisserie or corner café for something high-fat or high-sugar when you get to work. Gradually changing your eating habits starts with breakfast. Start small, an apple or banana, or a slice of toast, or start at the weekend with a breakfast that's a real treat for you and your family, perhaps melon and strawberries or warm muffins. Relax at breakfast and reflect on the day ahead, make it a time to read the paper. If you find this a problem, make it a goal.

A lunchtime sandwich is not enough to see you through the afternoon into the early evening: if this is all you eat, you will almost certainly hit a vulnerable patch and reach for poor-quality food. Avoid this by eating a good lunch. Remember that you can mix every kind of vegetable and most fruits into a salad. Don't be afraid to try new things – if you only like one in five then at least you have gained one new salad mix. If you start juicing you can make excellent dressings that are not smothered in oil.

If you have a staff restaurant, eat lots of carbohydrates, with fresh vegetables and fruits and maybe a slice or two of brown bread. If the food served is nutritionally poor, complain and hassle until something is done. To save time and money, and if you're out on the road, cook an extra portion the night before, or cook a couple of jacket potatoes while the evening meal is cooking. Even if you are busy at lunchtime, maybe with exercise, swimming, walking or shopping, it's important to make time to eat your lunch. NEVER SKIP IT. Evening meals are either a pleasurable experience or time of turmoil. If it is generally a sociable meal, possibly eaten quite late, you might find investing in a slow cooker allows you to make it a little earlier. You may hate this time of day – it's been a bad day, the children show no signs that they might be ready for bed, you're hungry and the last thing you want to do is get a meal. Start with a fresh juice, or some rice cakes and maybe a banana. A rice cooker comes into its own here, you can put it on and forget all about it while you decide what else to eat. Planning is particularly important for evening meals, simply because it is so easy to say 'I can't be bothered' and pick up a takeaway.

Snacks should provide you with energy. Good foods like fresh fruits, dried fruits, seeds, natural low fat yogurt (add fresh fruit), baps, pitta breads, sandwiches crammed full of fresh salad with chicken and fish are ideal to snack on. Try and eat as many different good foods as you can throughout the day. Aiming for variety ensures a good balance of carbohydrates, protein, vitamin, minerals and a little fat.

You may find you function best by snacking through the day on small amounts of good, energy-giving foods or you may prefer three straight meals. Most of us are somewhere in between. Use the diary to help you decide what works best for you.

There are suggestions for all meals and nutritious snacks throughout the diary – use these as a basis on which to work and experiment with your own flavours and combinations.

Fresh fruits and vegetables should form a MAJOR part of what you eat. Try anything you have not tried before. Sweet carrots juiced with fresh coriander and an orange taste wonderful and are a great way to get lots of vitamins and minerals inside your body.

It takes time to know what to look for when buying fruit and vegetables. Vegetables should be firm to the touch and crispy; make sure that onions, tomatoes, mushrooms, peppers and aubergines are not wrinkled or soft and that they have no damp patches or signs of bruising. Store all vegetables and salad in the drawer section of the fridge and make sure the drawer is dry.

The more vegetables you can eat raw, the better. Chop them into your salad, or juice them with a carrot or apple for sweetness. If you want them hot, invest in a steamer to preserve as many nutrients as possible.

Carbohydrates

About 60–70 per cent of your daily food intake should be carbohydrate. This is the best source of fuel for your body, high in energy and easy to burn. Carbohydrates themselves are not fattening, but when you smother them with rich, buttery sauces, you tip the balance from good burning fuel to saturated fuel, which is harder to burn and easier to store. Excess carbohydrate, simply cooked, is far less likely to be stored as fat (and, to be honest, it's quite difficult to eat excessive amounts of these extremely filling foods).

To avoid storage and encourage the burning of energy, divide your carbohydrate intake into 4–5 equal sized, regular snacks/meals during the day. Remember that eating high-quality carbohydrates satisfies your appetite and makes you less vulnerable to high-fat and high-sugar snacks.

Best sources

Pasta is full of goodness and is filling. Don't forget noodles, which are easy to cook and taste great with stir fry vegetables.

Potatoes are an excellent source of fuel but of course if you roast them in oil or smother them in butter or margarine they are fattening. Try roasting in a little water and rosemary or any other herbs you would like to try. Also try sweet potatoes (cook like jacket potatoes), roast parsnips, yams and plantain. Roast green bananas make a lovely dessert.

Rice is great tasting and brown is best, but try all kinds including risotto, basmati, and wild rice. All taste slightly different and they need to be cooked slightly differently.

Wholemeal bread has so much flavour that to spread fat on is really unnecessary. Bread is also extremely filling, so you don't need much to feel full. Health food shops often stock the best breads.

Cereals are generally under-rated. Include Weetabix, wheat flakes, muesli, shredded wheat, bran flakes, puffed wheat, whole grains, oats, millet, barley and corn. Avoid any thing with a high sugar content.

Useful gadgets and equipment

You may not be a gadget person, but there are definitely a few worth investing in. All make life easier and they do not have to cost the earth. Decide from the list here which you might find most useful – you can always add others later.

A vegetable peeler means that you remove only a thin layer of skin from vegetables, and don't throw half the goodness away.

A vegetable steamer that sits in your saucepan is inexpensive and easy to use. There are many variations on the market, some of which allow you to cook a whole meal in one pan. Steamed vegetables retain all their flavour and crispness, which can be lost with other cooking methods.

A salad spinner means goodbye to soggy lettuce. There are so many wonderful salad ingredients in the supermarkets today, and it is a pity to spoil them simply because you can't get lettuce dry enough.

My favourite – a **juicer**. What a great way to ensure you really do get your daily quota of five or more fruits and vegetables! It is impossible to describe the taste of freshly juiced fruit and vegetables. If you don't want to buy one straight away (they can be pricey), find someone who has one and ask to try it – your mind will be made up for you. (Unfortunately juicers come with an built-in problem – they are a real pain to clean, but if you wash it up immediately, it soon becomes a part of your daily routine.) Juices are great for getting over hunger pangs, good for starters while you prepare the rest of the meal (and stop you picking while you do so) and improve the look of your hair, skin and eyes.

A slow cooker means you can prepare tomorrow's meal while you are cooking today's, then you simply set the timer to be ready when you come home. It means that you do not stop off for a fast food meal or eat biscuits, nuts or crisps while you wait for a meal to cook. Alternatively invest in a terracotta oven pot, which cooks food in its own juices. Set the timer on the oven and come home to a cooked meal.

A microwave allows you to cook larger portions to freeze and use on 'I can't be bothered to cook' nights.

If you like bananas, which don't juice well, you may appreciate a **blender**, especially for frothy shakes using soya milk and apple juice. A blender is great for making sauces, soups and purées.

A rice cooker cooks perfect rice for one or ten in 20 minutes, then stops cooking and turns itself on to warm, and stays this way for up to two hours. Try adding a handful of raisins after it has stopped cooking – they swell up and taste delicious – or all sorts of herbs and spices.

Protein

Your body needs protein for growth and the formation of new tissues, and for repairing damaged tissues, but if you eat too much protein and are not extremely active, your body has difficulty using it as fuel and stores it as fat. Aim to make about 15–20 per cent of your daily intake protein.

Best sources

A lot of the best sources of protein tend to be high in saturated fats, so you have to decide how much fat you want to consume daily. Use beans or lentils to replace some or all of the meat in stews, casseroles and pies.

Low-fat dairy products, such as skimmed milk, cottage cheese, natural yogurt are good sources of protein, as is soya milk.

Eggs are good protein (go for free range), but the yolks contain cholesterol, so limit to a couple a week, or use the whites only.

White meats such as chicken and turkey, without skin, and fish (trout, cod, tuna or salmon, although this is high in fat too).

Brown bread and rice also contain protein.

FIRST STEPS TO FITNESS

Fat

We all need a certain amount of body fat for protection, cushioning and insulation around the organs; it also forms an essential part of the membranes which make up every cell in the body as well as the brain, nerves, tissues and bone marrow. Women need a little more than men to ensure normal hormonal and menstrual functions can occur. This does not mean rolls of fat – it means a good pinch.

If you eat good foods, you should be getting enough fat from your normal daily intake. All processed foods have fats and sugars added, so read labels carefully and don't be deceived by the big lettering saying 'low fat' (the food will contain more sugar; 'low sugar' usually means added fat). The recommended daily allowance of fat is between 10 and 30g a day, or 10–20 per cent of your total daily food intake.

AVOID OR CUT BACK ON

EAT MORE OF

AVOID OR CUT BACK ON	EAT MORE OF
Butter is pure animal fat, as are hydrogenated, all hardened fat spreads, margarines and other spreading fats. If you can't do without, try soya margarine, but make sure that it has not been chemically processed and spread it thinly.	Moisten bread with tomato purée, mustard, horseradish, cranberries, chopped tomatoes with spring onions, coriander and/or basil – improvise and invent.
All marbled meats (those white flecks are fat). Reduce beef, lamb, duck, pork. Cut all visible fat off before cooking. Choose lean cuts and buy the best you can afford.	Skinless turkey and chicken. Try Quorn occasionally.
Most cheeses are high in fat. Try to cut down – apart from anything else, you'll start to appreciate the flavour better if you eat it less often.	Lower-fat cheeses – Edam, ricotta, quark.
Full-fat milk.	Ease yourself gradually into semi-skimmed, then skimmed, or try soya milk sweetened with apple juice. Spinach, kale, broccoli, tofu and canned fish are all good alternative sources of calcium.
Fried foods.	Grilled, baked or steamed foods.
Fast-food takeaways are all high in fat. Limit to once a fortnight as an absolute maximum.	Try a new recipe – be adventurous. Most takeaways really are rather boring.
Cooking oils. Try halving what the recipe recommends – I guarantee you won't notice the difference.	Olive oil is the best you can buy. Use sparingly, but you deserve the best.
Convenience foods, with the sole exception of frozen vegetables. All processed foods have hidden fats, sugar and salt added to them. They are nutritionally poor and financially pricey. Stop buying them.	Fresh is best. You will burn more calories chopping vegetables (not to mention carrying them home) than opening the microwave and putting a convenience food inside. Different combinations of vegetables will make a huge difference to the quality of what you eat. Try them all.
Pastries, cakes, biscuits. Make your treats more in line with the new you – haircut, swimwear, underwear, something just for you.	The best alternative has to be fresh fruit. Bananas are sweet, easy to carry and full of energy. Don't overdose on one fruit – keep it

All breakfast cereals with added sugar.

varied. And, of course, most fruits are great juiced.

Corn/bran flakes, porridge, toasted wholemeal bread, wholemeal muffins, wholemeal pancakes with fresh chopped fruit and yogurt are all good breakfasts.

Jams and marmalades. Most contain less than 50 per cent fruit – the rest is sugar. Read the labels carefully.

If you need them (and you may if you're cutting down on butter and other spreads), seek out sugar-free. Some supermarkets do them, or try the health-food shop.

Fish canned in oil.

Tuna and salmon are excellent, but buy them canned in water or brine (which has salt added). Also buy fresh.

Bottled dressings and sauces.

Home made is best, as you know exactly what goes into the ingredients. Make up larger amounts and store in fridge or freezer for another day.

Refined foods of all descriptions are really not helping you to feel good about yourself. Drop one at a time and top up on carbohydrates so that you do not go hungry

Fresh ingredients simply cooked are going to make you look and feel better.

Breaking some addictions

Addictions are natural, but some people are better able to control them than others. A craving or addiction that becomes an obsession obviously needs specialist help, but for most of us, cravings or addictions are simply habits that with time and effort can be broken.

The reason addictions are so hard to break is that we are used to having what we want (hunger here has very little to do with it), so giving it up feels like a deprivation. Breaking a comfortable addiction does not mean that you will never be able to eat or drink something again, but it will make that food or drink special, a once a week, or once a month treat. (You may in any case find that as your tastebuds change and develop, you want whatever was your own particular weakness less often.)

I have been addicted to a greater or lesser extent at various times in my life to tea, coffee, chocolate and sugar. My parents constantly had the kettle on for tea, at all

hours of the day and night. I never even considered that I might be addicted – 10 or 15 cups a day, no problem. But of course there was: all that tea was preventing my body from absorbing the vitamins and minerals I needed from the food I was eating.

How to stop

First, try to identify the association between certain activities or places and the desire to drink coffee or tea or eat certain foods. You may not be aware that you are doing it, but if you mark it down in the diary you may well be able identify whether there is a trigger to your craving – time of day, certain person or situation – as well as how you perform on and react to these stimulants.

Look at what you are having in terms of 'comfort' food and drink. Do you really enjoy it, every single time? Is there is a pattern? Is it the time of day? The person you are with? Were you genuinely hungry? If you know what you are doing and why, you have the power of choice. You can choose not to have a biscuit, rather than reaching for one because it's four o'clock and you always have a biscuit at four o'clock. Take it slowly. Identify one trigger situation and make it a goal for a month or two. Just concentrate on the one situation that is giving you so much grief. It will gradually become a thing of the past.

How long will it take?

It takes at least four weeks to feel in control of stimulants. Coming off them may cause side effects, giving you a slight headache or a feeling of irritability as your body adapts. These feelings will slowly dissipate over the first 3–4 days if you stick with it.

Try some of the alternatives suggested and keep yourself occupied at trigger times: go for a walk, phone a friend, read a book, have a soak in the bath. Make sure that you eat sufficiently and frequently to ensure that you are not hungry, out of control, and looking for a quick fix.

Saying no

We all find ourselves going places and doing things that we don't want to, just because we are frightened, or unable, to say no.

But the more you practise saying it, the easier it rolls off the tongue. After a few times people soon get the message. I have had to ban friends from giving me chocolate, which I had great difficulty in doing, but slowly and gradually they got the hint. Now, if I'm lucky, I get flowers and I don't think about or miss the chocolates.

Always show appreciation to someone for their effort and for their offer, but if you really feel that you have had your quota for today or genuinely don't want it, say no. Each time you say so, you are confirming that you are in control, so congratulate yourself.

Coffee

Coffee gives an energy burst which is so shortlived that you are looking for your next hit within the hour. If you give in every time through the day, you need more and come down further after each initial buzz. You may be unable to eat regularly, your appetite is depressed, your insides are churned up and

you feel hyper, and possibly anxious. Then comes the feeling of irritability (maybe you don't notice but others almost certainly do). The net result is that you are tired, have no energy, yet do not sleep well.

If coffee is what you like, you will find it distressing to stop. Don't give up overnight but gradually, over the weeks try to reduce the number of cups you drink daily, easing down to one cup per day and drinking it at the time when you would most appreciate it. If you can reduce the number of cups you have in this way, you may eventually be able to make coffee a weekend treat. The first three days are the hardest, then you start to come to life.

Even decaffeinated coffee reduces your ability to absorb vital minerals, including iron. Most people, and women in particular, do not get enough iron, which makes you feel permanently drained. Shortage of iron also prevents other vitamins and minerals being absorbed properly.

Tea

Like coffee, tea is addictive. Although the caffeine content is minimal when compared with coffee (you have to have a really strong cup to compete), tea contains tannin which prevents the absorption of iron and zinc, both of which are important to the absorption of other vital vitamins and minerals, including vitamin C.

You may need to stop altogether for two to four weeks to break the addiction. Note what effect it is having on you over the weeks. The first three days are the hardest, only then does the craving start to lessen its grip on your body and mind.

Try herbal teas in a variety of flavours (you will quickly get bored if you stick to one). There are lots of variety packs on the market and many different makes – try them all, because they all taste so different. Be warned – some smell infinitely better than they taste. You may need some honey for sweetness to start with, but do try and wean yourself off this.

Sugar

The more you have, the more you want – that is a fact. Sugar is addictive because of its effect on our moods and our energy levels and is probably the most addictive stimulant, simply because it is everywhere you look. Don't be fooled by the technical terms – syrups, maltose, sucrose, glucose and honey are all sugars.

If you continue to consume so much sugar in the form of sweets, biscuits and cakes, you will never be able to shift any extra weight and you will be constantly craving and crying out for your sugar fix. Sugar affects us all differently: you may find your moods swing, you may become irritable, depressed, nervous, aggressive, suffer from headaches, be unable to concentrate, unable to sleep properly, unable to stop crying ... the list goes on. Think about yourself and how you personally react to sugar and note it in your diary. Is there a pattern?

Stop adding sugar to your drinks and your cereals and anything else you add it to. Use fresh or dried fruit as often as possible to gradually reduce your sugar intake. Don't despair if everything tastes sour to begin with – over the weeks this will become less acute.

Fresh and dried fruits are great sources of sweetness and good pick-me-ups. They do contain sugar, but in a natural form which gives a slower release of energy over a longer period of time. If you do suffer from periods of low energy, it's very important to eat a small amount of good food regularly, every three to four hours. This will help you to maintain an even blood sugar level (p. 29).

Carry fresh fruit with you at all times so that you are not hungry.

Alcohol

Most of us like a drink occasionally. Watch out, however, as alcohol will seriously contribute to your excess fat. Note in your diary how many drinks you have each day. The more you drink, the less appetite for food you have, so you drink more, accumulating more empty calories and less nutritious ones from good-quality foods. This has a terrible effect on the absorption of many vitamins and minerals, including vitamins C and the B complex, calcium, magnesium and zinc and, over time, it can have a devastating effect on your body.

Look for alternatives; try not drinking at all; or limit your intake to a couple of glasses a week. If this is a serious problem for you, get help – you are affecting your mental and physical performance for years to come. There are some great alternative non-alcoholic drinks on the market, so be adventurous and try something new.

Again this takes time and should be included in your goals and worked on over the weeks. I have gone from drinking almost daily, to just drinking occasionally and making that drink special, like champagne or a really good Belgian beer or two (yes, that's all it takes to feel jolly – it's amazing how your tolerance decreases when you stop drinking).

Chocolate

We learn to associate chocolate with self-indulgence and treats from the earliest age, and this is perpetuated into adulthood as we give and receive chocolates for all occasions.

The majority of chocolate on the shelves contains less than 30 per cent cocoa (the chocolate content); the rest is sugar and saturated fats. As a result, you may not actually be craving the chocolate, but the sugar and fat. Think about that.

Try buying chocolate that contains more than 30 per cent cocoa and consequently less sugar and fat, gradually easing your way into the real, fuller flavoured varieties.

If you don't want to cut it out (I certainly don't – I have chocolate every now and then, and don't feel guilty about it, I just wallow in the moment) be more choosy about when you have it and what you have. If you do want to stop altogether, start snacking on fresh fruit. Gradually your tastebuds will desire less sugar, so that over three to four weeks you should be over the longing for chocolate.

Cigarettes

I don't really need to tell you because you already know that smoking causes all sorts of problems and diseases, and can kill you.

Smoking affects your fitness level, suffocating the oxygenated cells that you breathe in which makes your workouts much harder, as you struggle to breathe. This, of course, makes activity less pleasurable and undermines your motivation because it all seems too difficult. You have to decide how important becoming fitter and healthier is to you.

There are many books and magazines that suggest various ways to stop smoking. Decide what and when might work for you. Make this one of your goals, but be sensible about it: if this habit has been part of your life for a long time, don't expect to quit quickly. Start by working out which situations are going to give you the most grief, and have a strategy for dealing with them – buy a yo-yo, go to the gym, get moving, the sooner you kick start your body, the sooner you will feel mentally able to deal with kicking this habit.

You may start to eat more to occupy your hands and mouth, so be prepared with good-quality nutricious snacks. Try to start a new hobby that keeps your hands busy. Constantly remind yourself why you are doing this, keep writing it in the diary.

Answering some questions

Q How long do I have to keep exercising?

A For ever – this is for life. This is why it is so important to try everything once, because you must enjoy what you are doing. There has to be a sense of fun to keep you going. If you vary your fitness activities as much as possible, you will enjoy getting and keeping fit even more. The ultimate benefit is an improved quality of life.

Aerobic work involves taking in larger quantities of oxygen than normal, either through brisk walking or cycling, or other aerobic activities. Maintaining a healthy heart and lungs to pump oxygen around to the working muscles allows you to be mobile and – best of all – makes you feel good.

Start to build your fitness level, now. Once you have achieved a level of fitness you are happy with, you can maintain it easily and keep your body fat down on three to five hours a week so long as you are eating well and keeping your energy levels high.

Q Is losing weight going to cure all my problems?

A Definitely not! But what it will do is give you the encouragement, strength and stamina (the ability to keep going) to gradually change things that you are not happy with. Losing body fat will make you feel better, enable you to be more mobile, allow you to reach a fitness level suitable to your busy lifestyle, and increase your self-esteem. Exercise will help you keep things under control, allow you to release tension and energize the muscles that have helped you through the day. It also boosts your metabolism to burn and use up all those excess calories you have eaten, for one reason or another.

Q Will exercise stop me feeling stressed out?

A Yes. We all suffer from stress at some time in our lives and we all have different tolerances to it: one person's unbearable strain is another's spur to get things done. The important thing is that you recognize in yourself when you are getting stressed, since prolonged stress can seriously damage your mental and physical health.

Most of your reactions to stress go unnoticed, but your muscles tense, your breathing becomes faster and shallower, you sweat more, your digestion slows, and you have feelings of anxiety, anger or frustration. The adrenalin keeps flowing and your pulse is pumping. If you do not release some of this built-up adrenalin, over a period of time your ability to sleep is affected. If you ignore signs of stress, you risk increased levels of the liver-releasing sugar, cholesterol, and fatty acids in the blood, which lead to high blood pressure and the possibility of stroke and heart attack.

The value of exercise in this can't be overemphasized. The sooner you realize that exercise makes you and your body feel better, the sooner you will feel able to deal with life's everyday tension builders. Do gentle rhythmic exercise, such as walking or swimming, try yoga or tai chi – there are many classes to choose from – or perhaps you need something more active to release tension.

Give yourself time to relax your whole body. Each day allow yourself at least 10 minutes to relax, maybe in the bath or taking the dog for a walk, or treat yourself to a massage. We spend money on clothes to wear, and yet they look terrible if you are tense and angry. Your body needs you to care for it and to pamper it, it needs time out. Your clothes will hang better and your whole body image, presence and posture will improve as you become more relaxed.

If you lose control, take long deep breaths in, and breathe them out slowly, several times. If someone angers you while you are driving, stop the car, and take a minute to relax, breathe deeply, try to smile – it's amazing how much better it makes you feel.

Q Why do my muscles turn to fat when I stop exercising?

A Put simply, they don't. Fat and muscle are different substances with specific and separate functions. Muscles cover your skeleton to support it; fat covers your muscles to insulate and protect them. Fat cells are designed to store fat; muscles, by contrast, are responsible for developing force to create movement, allowing you to move about and stand upright. If you stop or reduce your fitness training, your muscles shrink in size, they do not turn to fat. If you continue to eat in excess of your daily requirement – which drops considerably if you stop or reduce your daily activities and fitness training – the fat cells in and around the muscles multiply to accommodate the excess calories that you have consumed.

Q How many abdominal curls must I do a day to reduce the fat on my stomach?

A Sorry, no can do! No matter how many you do daily, you will not reduce the levels of body fat accumulated here. The underlying muscles of the abdomen will get a better tone and become firmer to the touch, but the layers of fat will still wobble over the top and may feel even looser than usual because of the firmness underneath.
The only way to get rid of body fat is to eat good, energy-giving foods that you will burn easily and get moving to increase your metabolism and encourage your body to burn fat.

Q No pain, no gain, true or false?

A It depends what you mean by pain. Shutting your finger in the door or burning yourself – that's pain, real throbbing uncontrollable pain. During exercise you have to ask your body to work a bit harder, in order to experience an overload. Your body gets you through your normal day-to-day activities without overloading, so when you start to challenge it to improve your fitness level, you will feel some discomfort. But with each challenge – one more repetition, one more minute's walk – your body is building strength. When you feel a little discomfort, this is a sign that you have reached the overload and are working at the right level of intensity. Of course if you are feeling real pain during exercise, stop straight away and check that you are doing everything correctly – and that includes your posture.

Q About 48 hours after exercise I'm unable to move because it's so

painful. Why?

Ⓐ You have done too much too soon. You have used muscles or groups of muscles that have not felt any kind of regular overload recently. This sort of overload causes microscopic tears in the fibres which make up your muscles. If you continue to exercise gently, the pain should ease off after about 24 hours.

If, however, you continue to feel real pain, or are badly bruised, or unable to move, lift or push, you have caused those microscopic tears to become inflamed and swell within the muscle. Pain of this type should ease off over the course of three or four days, but if it continues, you should attend a sports injury clinic.

You can and should at all costs avoid this happening. Ease yourself into exercise slowly.

Ⓠ **Should I exercise when I have a cold, or feel a bit under the weather?**

Ⓐ When you are not in top condition, your body's immune system has to work overtime to try to correct whatever imbalance in your body is making you feel ill. Use this time as a rest period to allow your body to heal itself. If you insist on exercising, you are asking your body to do two major things, first deal with whatever is wrong and, second, burn up lots of energy that your immune system could be using to make you fit and well. After time off, ease yourself back into your regime gently. Start again at a lower level than you left off – for if you don't you are certain to drain the body of its energy and it could lead to injury.

Ⓠ **Should I work out through an injury?**

Ⓐ Definitely not. Always get an injury checked out, do not ignore it and hope that it will go away. If you continue to work, without allowing it to heal, you will aggravate any injury. Strapping up is not the answer. It's OK to strap up for support, but strapping an injury to allow you to get through a workout will simply put strain on your other muscles and

could lead to permanent damage. When you have an injury treated, ask what stretches you should do, how often you should do them and how long you should hold them. When you have done all the necessary stretching to help the muscle back to its normal range of movement, you can resume exercise, easing yourself into it gently and taking particular care not to aggravate or injure the damaged area. It can take weeks, months, even years to heal an injury, so take care of this area.

Ⓠ **What are the pelvic floor muscles?**

Ⓐ The pelvis connects the upper body to the lower body and it facilitates most movement in the lower body. In women it also protects the uterus, bladder and, in pregnancy, the foetus.

Forming the floor of this basin is a hammock, a sling of muscles called the pelvic floor muscles. Around the openings, in men and women, there are extra loops of muscle which contract to keep the openings tightly closed when you put pressure on your abdomen by laughing, coughing or sneezing when your bladder is full. Strong pelvic muscles stop your bladder leaking in these situations (the technical term is stress incontinence) and are vital in pregnancy to avoid such problems later, but they also improve the quality of your sex life.

Regular exercise of your pelvic floor muscles can avoid stress incontinence, which can strike people who have not even had a baby, as young as 30. Start with your posture. Stand tall, gently pulling in your lower abdominal muscles. You should be able to feel your pelvic floor muscles contracting too. Now you have located them, you can start work on them. Sit, stand or lie. Imagine you are a building and your pelvic floor muscles are a lift. Tighten the muscles around the back and front passages as if closing the lift doors tightly. Now tighten a little more as if you are taking the lift to the second floor. Tighten more as if to reach the third floor, continue until you reach as far as you can go, hold for few seconds, then gradually descend again to ground floor and gently pull up to stop on the ground floor. Repeat this as often as you can during the day.

Above all, take your time – it is always better to do 20 well than 50 badly. Quality does count.

Q What exactly is my blood sugar level? How does it affect me?

A It's part of the daily juggling act. Keeping your blood sugar level even throughout the day will allow you to keep hunger at bay, which means weight loss becomes less of an issue – if you are not hungry, you won't eat too much of the wrong foods. Glucose (blood sugar) in your bloodstream enables your body's cells to make energy. When the level of blood sugar drops, your body signals that it is hungry. If you ignore these initial signals, your body will relay them to you in other ways: you may feel drowsy, nervous, irritable, unable to concentrate, or you may get a headache. In extreme cases you may be nauseous or dizzy.

Is this your day (or similar to it)? You wake in the morning and it takes you at least 15 minutes to be alert. Your body needs energy, which you take as a signal that you need coffee, tea, cigarettes, sugar on your cereal, biscuits. You have your fix and are ready for the world, but around 10 or 11 am, you get that hungry, tired, lethargic feeling. So you have another fix of your breakfast 'pick-me-up', and on to lunch after which you feel sleepy and in an ideal world would have a siesta. By the end of working day (probably with another couple of coffees or teas and a few biscuits to get you through the afternoon) you are drained,

much too tired to contemplate exercising. With luck, you'll get home, feed the children, then fall asleep in front of the TV with a blinding headache. And so to bed for a restless night.

If you recognize one or more of these feelings, your body may have a blood sugar imbalance and you need to look at your eating habits, both in terms of what you eat and how often you eat. Once you recognize that you do need to redress your daily food intake, your levels of concentration and your energy will increase, as will your feelings that you are in control.

To have the energy to start exercising and gain some control over your life, you need to cut out or drastically reduce your intake of simple (that is, processed) sugars – chocolate, biscuits, cakes and sugars (glucose, maltose), all of which have a profound effect on your blood sugar level. The more you eat wholemeal breads (why not try rye or pumpernickel), wholemeal pasta and rice, pulses, vegetables and fruits, the easier you will find it regulate your blood sugar level and avoid the peaks and troughs that make you reach for low-energy, low-goodness foods.

Ready?

This is where you start on the road to a new, fitter, healthier you. But before you do anything else, take a look through the week's diary and try to decide when you are going to do your walking and your exercises. I find it best to work first thing in the morning so that I don't have to worry about finding time later in the day, but you can work at any time that suits you best. When do you have most energy? Think about it and write the time you are going to exercise down in the diary. It may be a bit of a struggle to find both the time and the energy to get started on week one, but I promise you it will be worth it when you do.

You will also notice as you look through the week's diary that there is space for you to record what you eat during the day. I've added a suggestion that you might consider each day, to get you thinking along the right lines, but you should write down honestly what you eat and when. There is also space for you to note your goals for the day and the week. This is because we are all different, so individual targets are going to differ. I've also added some tips to help you achieve those goals. And there is space for you to record how you feel (see pp. 12–13): does exercise make you feel better? Did you feel great after climbing the stairs rather than using the lift? Was it hard work, or surprisingly easy to resist a biscuit?

By the end of this first week, you will be walking five minutes a day comfortably. As you build up toward that magical five minute mark over the week, you will be taking in oxygen and distributing it around your body to your working muscles and your brain. This has several effects. Firstly, oxygen can in itself give you a natural high so that you start to feel better about yourself and more able to cope with the strains and stresses of everyday life. And, since your heart is one of the muscles circulating the oxygen around your body, it beats more strongly, which has to be good news for your health. Finally, all this muscle work burns calories, which means that you should lose body fat.

This week you will also start on your first exercise, the rather ominous-sounding wall press. This simple exercise, which can be done almost anywhere, is designed to strengthen your chest, shoulders and the backs of your arms. It's very easy to neglect the upper body, but it is important to have some strength here since we all do our fair share of carrying heavy bags and lifting children. You may not have problems now, but as you get older a neglected upper body can cause pain in your lower back, shoulders and neck and – eventually – restricted movement in these areas. All of which mean that is worthwhile making an effort now.

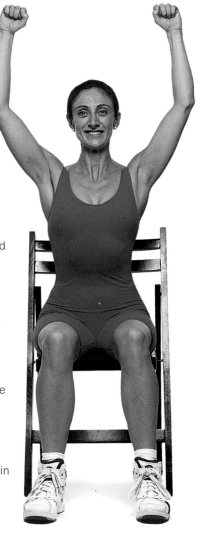

We'll start with just one set of up to six repetitions (do as many as you can comfortably with good technique). This needs to be done twice during the week, but leave 48 hours between these sessions so that you don't work the same muscles on consecutive days. If you are going to walk and do the wall presses at the same time of day, walk first so that your body is already taking in some of the extra oxygen your muscles are going to need for the strength exercise.

Away you go and good luck!

WALL PRESS

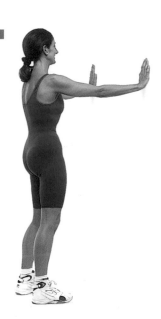

1

Warm up and stretch.

Stand facing and about 60 cm (2 ft) away from a wall, with your legs slightly more than hip width apart – you should feel comfortable.

Pull in your lower abdomen and lift your ribcage.

Relax your shoulders and look forward.

Place your hands on the wall at about the same height as your chest and slightly wider apart than your shoulders. You're now ready.

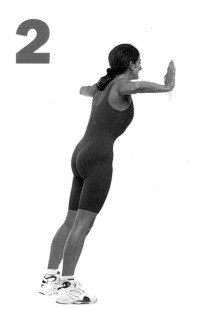

2

Focus on the area you are going to be working – your chest, shoulders and the backs of your arms.

Breathe in as you bend your elbows and press into the wall.

Pause, then breathe out as you use the muscles of your arms and chest to press away from the wall. Make your muscles do the work and take your time – each repetition should take you about four seconds.

CHEST STRETCH

1

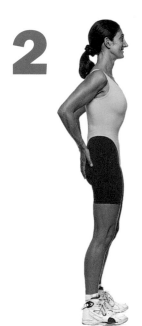

This exercise will stretch the muscles across the front of your chest.

Breathe normally throughout.

Standing with your back straight, pull in your tummy. Lift your ribcage and relax your shoulders.

Slightly soften the pressure in your knees, so that they do not lock. By doing this, your pelvis will be tilted forward so that it is in line with your body.

2

Placing your hands on your buttocks and relaxing your shoulders, very gently move your elbows in towards each other, bringing the shoulder blades together and opening up the chest.

Hold the stretch for 8 - 10 seconds when you warm up, for 20 - 30 seconds as part of your cool down, then relax.

Fitness for the day

0–2 min walk

Use this walk to get your whole body moving. Stand tall, roll your shoulders back, down and round to relax and loosen your neck and shoulder area. Keep your back straight and your chest and ribcage high, and pull in your tummy muscles. Start to take control of your body, breathe in and feel the oxygen circulating to your muscles, helping you to get your body (and mind) in gear. Be proud of yourself: you deserve to be.

★ Fitness goal

If you can't decide, walk one stop before you get the bus or train.

FEELING SCALE FOR EXERCISE

20 MAXIMUM EXERTION

19 EXTRA HARD

17 VERY HARD

16 HARDER

15 HARD

12 LIGHT

10 VERY LIGHT

Food for the day

Breakfast

2 Weetabix with milk + little sugar / tea

Snack

Lunch

Jacket potato bursting with

tuna and sun-dried tomatoes

Brown bread sandwich little goat cheese + salad

Snack 4 slices melon + apple

Noodles, stir fried veg

Evening meal

Light snack

★ Goal for the week

Remember what you were thinking as you took a good hard look at yourself, then decide.

Mood for the day

Mood at the start of the day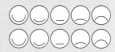

Mood at the end of the day

Food tips

Forget any recipes that call for more than 30 ml (1 tablespoon) of oil or 30g (1 oz) of butter.

Motivation tips

Enjoy your exercise time as time for yourself. This is your indulgence for the day.

Fitness for the day

2 min walk

Enjoy the sensation of movement as you walk. Breathe in deeply and exhale slowly. When you have finished your walk, take time to stretch your leg muscles.

This is a big day, with your first step on the way to putting some strength into your upper body. This will not give you huge muscles, but it will improve the appearance of your chest and the backs of your arms. It also strengthens your skeleton, helping it to support your internal organs and improving your posture.

Keep your torso stiff to ensure that your technique is correct and that you are protecting your lower back from injury. Think about the muscles you are working.

★ Food goal

If you can't decide, how about having one less cup of coffee, tea, glass of wine or beer?

Exercise 1: Wall press
0–6 reps, 1 set

FEELING SCALE FOR EXERCISE

20
MAXIMUM EXERTION

19
EXTRA HARD

17
VERY HARD

16
HARDER

15
HARD

12
LIGHT

10
VERY LIGHT

Food for the day

Breakfast _2x weetabix + tea_

Wholemeal pancakes with fruit salad and low-fat fromage frais

Snack
1 round brown sandwhich

Lunch _2 satseumas_
Banana

Snack _2 hmade fish cakes + stir fry veg_

Evening meal

Pear/Satsuma

Light snack

★ Goal for the week

How's it going?

Mood for the day

Mood at the start of the day

Mood at the end of the day

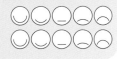

Fitness tips

Think of all the activities you can do when you feel better.

Motivation tips

Keep your immediate goals simple: taking one step at a time is better than five one day and none the next.

Fitness for the day
Walk 2–3 mins

Let's up the pace a little today. Stand tall, keep your lower abdomen pulled in and your ribcage lifted and concentrate on striding out. Make each stride a good one. Place your heel on the ground first, then the ball of your foot. Focus on your foot, then muscles of your leg, right from your toes through to your buttocks, feeling each step and making each step count.

When you have finished your walk, take time to stretch your leg muscles.

★ Fitness goal
How about ringing the local gym to ask about classes and sessions?

FEELING SCALE FOR EXERCISE

20
MAXIMUM EXERTION

19
EXTRA HARD

17
VERY HARD

16
HARDER

15
HARD

12
LIGHT

10
VERY LIGHT

Food for the day
Breakfast

Snack

Lunch

Snack
Low-fat yogurt with fresh fruit

Evening meal

Light snack

★ Goal for the week
Are you on course to achieve it?

Mood for the day
Mood at the start of the day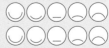

Mood at the end of the day

Food tips
Eat before you shop. If you shop on an empty stomach, you will buy all sorts of things you don't want.

Motivation tips
We all have our bad days. If you slide, don't dwell on it. Start again tomorrow.

Fitness for the day

Walk 3 mins

Are you really striding out? Concentrate on placing your feet, not stamping them down. When you have finished your walk, take time to stretch your leg muscles and if you are feeling good and can comfortably spare another couple of minutes, do so and congratulate yourself afterward.

Take your time with the wall presses so that each repetition really counts and each one is fully under control. Remember a repetition should take about four seconds. To get the timing right, you might find it helps to count 'one two' as you press into the wall and 'three four' as you press away. Did you find it OK? Too hard? If you found it difficult, remember that it's better to do four repetitions well than six badly. Don't cheat: you are only cheating yourself.

Exercise 1: Wall press
0–6 reps, 2 sets

FEELING SCALE FOR EXERCISE

20 MAXIMUM EXERTION

19 EXTRA HARD

17 VERY HARD

16 HARDER

15 HARD

12 LIGHT

10 VERY LIGHT

Food for the day

Breakfast

Snack

Lunch

Snack

Evening meal
Seafood and vegetable stir fry, with Thai spices

Light snack

★ Goal for the week
Are you still on course?

★ Food goal
If you failed the last one, try it again today.

Mood for the day

Mood at the start of the day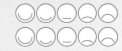

Mood at the end of the day

Fitness tips
Remind yourself how good you felt today after your walk – wasn't it worth it?

Motivation tips
Remember the three Ds – Desire, Drive, Dedication. You can do it.

Fitness for the day
3–4 mins

If you want to burn calories as you walk, it's important to use your arms as well as your legs. Let them swing freely from your shoulders. Bend your elbows slightly and keep your hands relaxed and start to pump – not swing – your arms. Pump up towards your chin in front, but keep your hands at around hip level on the down movement: don't push them too far back.

Using the muscles of your upper body, as well as those of your lower body, in your walking, keeps the movement controlled. And the more muscles you use, the harder your heart has to work to circulate blood and oxygen to those muscles. All this boosts the rate at which you convert oxygen into energy, which burns calories. It's that simple: the more calories you burn, the more body fat you lose.

When you have finished your walk, take time to stretch your leg muscles.

FEELING SCALE FOR EXERCISE

20 MAXIMUM EXERTION

19 EXTRA HARD

17 VERY HARD

16 HARDER

15 HARD

12 LIGHT

10 VERY LIGHT

Food for the day

Breakfast

Snack

Lunch

Snack
Cereal bar – check the health-food shops, theirs are usually the best. Watch the fat and sugar content

Evening meal

Light snack

★ Goal for the week
Are you still on target, or might you have been over-ambitious?

★ Fitness goal
How is it going?

Mood for the day

Mood at the start of the day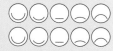

Mood at the end of the day

Food tips
Buy a smaller dinner plate. You will have the psychological advantage of a whole plateful, but will be eating less.

Motivation tips
Stick with it – you're doing brilliantly.

Fitness for the day
Walk 4 mins

Are you feeling positive about your walking now? Each day you should be standing a little taller and feeling a little better.

Remember to keep your ribcage lifted so that your diaphragm can function properly and your lungs have room to expand as they take in oxygen. Enjoy breathing, be conscious of inhaling and exhaling.

★ Food goal
To savour every mouthful – goals are more likely to be fulfilled if you keep them simple.

FEELING SCALE FOR EXERCISE

20 MAXIMUM EXERTION

19 EXTRA HARD

17 VERY HARD

16 HARDER

15 HARD

12 LIGHT

10 VERY LIGHT

Food for the day

Breakfast
An enormous bowl of fresh fruit salad

Snack

Lunch

Snack

Evening meal

Light snack

★ Goal for the week
Keep it up – you're almost there!

Mood for the day
Mood at the start of the day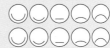

Mood at the end of the day

Fitness tips
When it gets difficult, visualize the body you want to achieve. Won't that make all your effort worthwhile?

Motivation tips
You have already taken the biggest step by facing the fact that you want to change your lifestyle.

Fitness for the day
Walk 5 mins

Well done. Five minutes' brisk walking is quite an achievement. You should feel great. More importantly, you have laid the foundations for the future, by making time in your daily schedule for exercise.

If you find you are breathless as you walk, reduce the length of your stride and keep your arms down for a few steps. Then, when your breathing is back to normal, gradually increase the pace and the pumping action of your arms.

★ Fitness goal
If you can't decide, walk one stop before you get the bus or train.

FEELING SCALE FOR EXERCISE

20 MAXIMUM EXERTION

19 EXTRA HARD

17 VERY HARD

16 HARDER

15 HARD

12 LIGHT

10 VERY LIGHT

Food for the day

Breakfast

Snack

Lunch

Snack

Evening meal

Light snack
Baked beans on toast

★ Goal for the week
Have you achieved your week's goal? If you have, well done, if not, perhaps you were being unrealistic. Pick one you can achieve and try again next week.

Food tips
If you're eating bread and jam, choose brown bread and sugar-free jam and miss out the layer of fat between the two. After a couple of weeks you won't even notice that those redundant calories are not there.

Mood for the day

Mood at the start of the day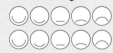

Mood at the end of the day

Motivation tips
Do something you enjoy when you're feeling vulnerable - but don't hit the biscuit tin.

WEEK TWO INTRODUCTION

This week, stride out as you aim to increase your daily walk from 5 to 10 minutes. Get your body moving, feel your temperature rising, enjoy that sensation of the wind in your face, think tall and positively – look forward to your walks as time for you. Finding the time might still be a problem, but if you stick with it, you will soon find walking fits into your lifestyle.

For this week's exercise, I have chosen to start focusing on the fronts of the thighs. There are four muscles here, which work in cooperation. Generally, the two smaller ones of the group are underworked; these run along the inner thigh, down to just above the knee. It's easy to see why this should be so, since most of our movements are forward or backward – rarely do we move sideways, extending the range of movement here.

Over time, as these muscles weaken, stress is put on your kneecaps, which can lead to pain and inflammation to the underside of the kneecap. You may notice this if you start jogging or step classes, or you may suffer with it when you climb stairs (is this another reason why you head for the lift?). As usual, a weakness in one area sets up a chain reaction as you transfer your weight away from the stressed area, which can lead to other injuries, not simply in your legs but throughout the body.

The leg extension will enable you to move and exercise without injury, and will greatly improve the shape of your thighs, making them appear leaner and more toned (and making knobbly knees less apparent). We're not talking bulk here; we are talking leaner and firmer. Increasing your strength in this area evens the stress distribution over the muscles, making aches and pains elsewhere less likely.

Be warned before you start, however, that it can take a long time before you see vast improvements in the shape of your legs. For a start, the legs are very strong – they need to be to carry you around all day (especially if you are carrying excess body weight). And, if you are carrying excess body fat, then quite a lot of it is likely to be in this area. It probably took you several years to build up the stores here, so it is going to take a lot more than 30 minutes walking daily to get rid of them. It needs exercises like the leg extension and it needs you to stop putting more fats and sugars inside you to go into the fat stores that are already there. Think of this as the start of a long tunnel: there really is light at the end, but it is going to take a while to get there. Don't worry about how long it's going to take, just have fun along the way.

LEG EXTENSION

Leg extensions are best done when you are sitting so that your back and torso are stable, and you can focus on just using the muscles at the fronts of your thighs. Take your time, making a conscious effort to enjoy and appreciate what the exercise is doing for you. You may find it helps to put on some good music with a slow beat and visualize how your thighs are going to look in future.

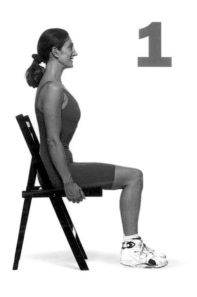

1 Warm up and stretch. Remember that warming up activates the fluid behind the knee that cushions the connecting bones of the upper and lower leg.

Sit with your back straight, ribcage lifted and tummy muscles pulled in. Hold on to the sides of your chair for added support. Keep your knees close together and in line with your hips.

Curl your toes toward your shins. Take a deep breath in and, as you breathe out, press upward, through the heel of your right foot, slowly extending your right leg upward, while keeping the back of your thigh in contact with the chair.

2 Extend your leg fully, but stop slightly short of locking your knee. Gently hold, squeezing deep into the muscle around the knee, holding on full extension for one second.

Breathe in as, leading with the heel of your foot, you lower back to the start position. Make sure you keep your thigh muscles slightly contracted so that you use the air as a resistance all the way down.

Work the stated number of repetitions, then repeat using your left leg. Work the stated number of reps and sets with both legs.

FRONT OF THIGH STRETCH

1 While some of you will find this exercise to be quite simple, others will have difficulty reaching and holding the ankle. Should this be the case, take hold of the cuff of your sock, legging, or jogging trousers.

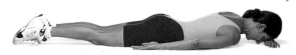

Lying face down, place your resting hand under your forehead for comfort. Ensure that your head is aligned with the spine and that your chin is facing downwards.

Keep your tummy pulled in and your hips firmly on the ground.

2 Gently ease your heel toward your buttocks, holding your ankle or sock with your working hand. Keep your knees together and the front of your thighs touching the ground.

Hold the stretch for 8–10 seconds when you warm up, for 20–30 seconds as part of your cool down, then relax.

Repeat with your other leg.

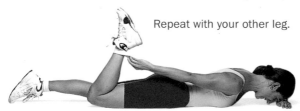

Fitness for the day
Walk 5 mins

Today you have a new exercise – the leg extension. Take your time, look at the photographs, focus on the coaching points and mentally feel the exercise. It is so good for the front of the thighs, where it is vital to build some strength to protect your knees from injury. Continue to check the photographs and coaching points to ensure good technique, take your time and do them slowly.

Exercise 1: Wall press
6–8 reps, 2 sets
Exercise 2: Leg extension,
4–6 reps, 1 sets

FEELING SCALE FOR EXERCISE

20
MAXIMUM
EXERTION
☐

19
EXTRA
HARD
☐

17
VERY
HARD
☐

16
HARDER
☐

15
HARD
☐

12
LIGHT
☐

10
VERY
LIGHT
☐

Food for the day

Breakfast

Snack

Lunch
Homemade fresh vegetable soup. Cook the night before, whizz in the blender, then microwave

Snack

Evening meal

Light snack

★ Goal for the week
A new one? Or something different? The choice is yours, but fill it in for every day.

★ Food goal
Repeat one of last week's if you didn't make it.

Mood for the day

Mood at the start of the day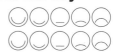

Mood at the end of the day

Fitness tips
Extend your stride, feel all your leg muscles working, and working well.

Motivation tips
The word 'can't' has no validity – at least 9 times out of 10 you can.

Fitness for the day
Walk 5–6 mins

An extra minute today! Extend your stride, enjoy yourself, breathe in some fresh air. Keep your abdominals pulled in, lower first, then upper, and finally lift your ribcage so that your chest and lungs can expand. Enjoy the sensation of being outside. If you're finding it difficult, slow down, ease yourself in gradually, make sure you are breathing comfortably. Have you got your whole body warm?

★ Fitness goal
The choice is endless – why not make it something that helps you reach this week's goal?

FEELING SCALE FOR EXERCISE

20 MAXIMUM EXERTION

☐

19 EXTRA HARD

☐

17 VERY HARD

☐

16 HARDER

☐

15 HARD

☐

12 LIGHT

☐

10 VERY LIGHT

☐

Food for the day

Breakfast

Snack

Lunch

Snack

Low-fat cottage cheese and sliced mango sandwich, using wholemeal or granary bread – exotic and delicious

Evening meal

Light snack

★ Goal for the week
Keep at it.

Food tips
Take snacks with you – a sandwich, dried fruit, mixed unsalted nuts, fresh fruit or juice, cereal bars. In this way, you won't be tempted by crisps and other savoury snacks, chocolate or biscuits when you feel hunger pangs.

Mood for the day

Mood at the start of the day
Mood at the end of the day

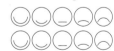

Motivation tips
Learn to say no.

Fitness for the day
Walk 6 mins

Aim for 8 reps of the wall press, but don't get disheartened if 7 is your limit. Take your time and enjoy the sensation of using and working your body. Likewise, aim for 6 Leg extensions and go for the 2 sets – you can do it, if you take it gently. Remember that the second set is always easier as your brain knows you can do it and your muscles are familiar with what you are asking them to do. Take it slowly and really feel your muscles working.

Exercise 1: Wall press
6–8 reps, 2 sets
Exercise 2: Leg extension
4–6 reps, 2 sets

FEELING SCALE FOR EXERCISE

20 MAXIMUM EXERTION
☐

19 EXTRA HARD
☐

17 VERY HARD
☐

16 HARDER
☐

15 HARD
☐

12 LIGHT
☐

10 VERY LIGHT
☐

Food for the day

Breakfast

Snack

Lunch

Snack

Evening meal

Light snack
Wholemeal pitta pockets filled with hummus and salad

★ Goal for the week
I'm sure you can do it!

Mood for the day
Mood at the start of the day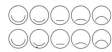
Mood at the end of the day

★ Food goal
To buy one exotic new fruit.

Fitness tips
Try a new activity, such as roller skating or hill climbing.

Motivation tips
Face up to what is stopping you living as you want – only you can change it.

WEEK TWO DAY FOUR

Fitness for the day
Walk 6–7 mins

Make time for the extra minute today. Concentrate on using your whole leg and feel all your leg muscles working. Keep your back straight and walk tall, look around and relax into the stride – not too relaxed though! Results take effort that only you can make. You need to keep the pace up in order to work aerobically, but be sure to increase your pace gradually.

★ Fitness goal
If you can't think of one, take a walk round the park at lunchtime.

FEELING SCALE FOR EXERCISE

20
MAXIMUM EXERTION

19
EXTRA HARD

17
VERY HARD

16
HARDER

15
HARD

12
LIGHT

10
VERY LIGHT

Food for the day
Breakfast
Summer porridge – oats with a couple of bananas, topped with the juice of a handful of strawberries

Snack

Lunch

Snack

Evening meal

Light snack

★ Goal for the week
Are you on course to achieve it?

Food tips
Each week buy one product you have not tried before – sundried tomatoes, couscous, lentils, brown rice. if you only like one of them, you have at least added that to your repertoire.

Mood for the day
Mood at the start of the day
Mood at the end of the day

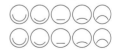

Motivation tips
Look at the jacket/skirt/trousers you want to wear. You will get there.

WEEK TWO DAY FIVE

Fitness for the day
Walk 7 mins

You may be feeling the effects of the last few days' exercises and walks, but don't worry. This slight soreness will fade away, and you will feel good from all the effort you have made. Remember all the reasons you are doing this.

Are your shoes comfortable? If you are feeling soreness around your shins, you may need new shoes. Check the heels, backs and insoles. And be sure to warm up properly.

★ Food goal
Work toward five servings of fruit or vegetables a day.

FEELING SCALE FOR EXERCISE

20 MAXIMUM EXERTION

19 EXTRA HARD

17 VERY HARD

16 HARDER

15 HARD

12 LIGHT

10 VERY LIGHT

Food for the day

Breakfast

Snack

Lunch

Snack

Evening meal
Rice with grilled or poached chicken and lots of vegetables

Light snack

★ Goal for the week
How are you doing?

Mood for the day

Mood at the start of the day

Mood at the end of the day

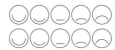

Fitness tips
Walk tall, think tall.

Motivation tips
Only you are in control. Take charge now.

Fitness for the day
Walk 7–8 mins

Get used to walking slightly faster and more upright than you are accustomed to – this extra pace is important. It may be a bit difficult, but hang in there. Try slowing down a little, get your breathing regular, then increase the pace again. Remember as you walk to lead with your heel and roll through to the ball of your foot. Keep your heels down and stand up straight.

★ Fitness goal
If you can't decide, how about walking an extra minute or two, really enjoying the sensation of movement?

FEELING SCALE FOR EXERCISE

20
MAXIMUM EXERTION

19
EXTRA HARD

17
VERY HARD

16
HARDER

15
HARD

12
LIGHT

10
VERY LIGHT

Food for the day
Breakfast

Snack
Mixed nuts (unsalted) and dried fruit, with plenty of water to drink

Lunch

Snack

Evening meal

Light snack

★ Goal for the week
Almost there?

Mood for the day
Mood at the start of the day

Mood at the end of the day

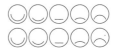

Food tips
Once a week treat yourself to your weakness – nothing is banned forever. You'll feel better for it.

Motivation tips
We all have bad days, don't worry about it.

Fitness for the day
Walk 9–10 mins

Well done! You have introduced another full 5 minutes exclusively for yourself into your day. I hope you're feeling proud of yourself – you should be. What a great feeling as you go into week three. Watch those fats and sugars and keep filling in your food diary.

★ Food goal
To say no to what you really do not want.

FEELING SCALE FOR EXERCISE

20
MAXIMUM
EXERTION
☐

19
EXTRA
HARD
☐

17
VERY
HARD
☐

16
HARDER
☐

15
HARD
☐

12
LIGHT
☐

10
VERY
LIGHT
☐

Food for the day

Breakfast

Snack

Lunch

Jacket potato filled with low-fat cheese, chopped onions and snipped chives

Snack

Evening meal

Light snack

★ Goal for the week
Did you make it – well done!

Mood for the day

Mood at the start of the day

Mood at the end of the day

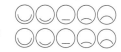

Fitness tips
Each day you are getting stronger, remember that.

Motivation tips
Knowing yourself and your body is the route to success.

WEEK THREE INTRODUCTION

Into the third week you go. You should be smiling at yourself, feeling good from within. You have, from nothing, built up and are incorporating a good 10 minutes walking into your daily lifestyle. Brilliant!

This week you are going to walk 10 minutes every day so that you know that doing this is never going to be a problem for you, but simply a natural part of what you do each day. Walk with vigour, let those arms do some work, get them up above your heart, make your walk more aerobic, make your heart work harder to get stronger, encourage your body to burn more fat. I know it feels alien to be pumping your arms, especially if you're used to walking slouched over with your shoulders forward and arms tucked in. But your self-consciousness will ease over the coming weeks, as you get into the stride and pattern of things, and your self-esteem starts to skyrocket. This will spill out into the rest of your life. Good posture gives you positive body language: walk tall and be proud of your achievements.

How are your moods in the morning? Are you a little more alert? Are you getting enough sleep? Continue to monitor your moods not only in the morning and at night, but note how you feel prior to exercise and again afterward. Is there a difference? Keeping a record will really help you to get in touch with how you feel.

Work hard on the two previous exercises; keep referring to the photographs and the coaching points each time you do them to be sure you are doing them correctly. Work slowly and focus on the muscles you are using.

Also this week, you are going to start working on the abdominal area, with an exercise for the lower abdominals. These are underused and their importance to your well-being vastly under estimated. You don't simply need good abdominal muscles to have a flat stomach (although that's what most of us – male and female – want); you need them also to ensure that your back has the help it needs to support your spine, and support and protect all your valuable organs.

Carrying excess weight around your abdomen can cause all sorts of problems for your back and hips. When you don't do any strength exercises for this area, the abdominal muscles become weak and those of the lower back even weaker. This can lead to anything from neck ache to severe pain of the lower back and into the hips and down the legs ... need I go on?

There is definitely an art to this exercise, so take your time and make the effort to get it right. Really think about and visualize the muscles at work.

LOWER ABDOMEN RAISE

1

Warm up and stretch, with lots of reaching and lifting from your waist and turning to right and left, while keeping your hips square to the front.

Lie with your back firmly pressed into the floor. Keeping your knees together, extend your legs out slightly. Make sure that your back stays firmly on the floor.

Your arms are not going to help you with this exercise, so relax them wherever is most comfortable for you – above your head, out to your sides, under your head, down by your hips.

Relax your legs: concentrate on total relaxation from your knees to your toes, focus your attention on your lower abdomen, picture the muscles deep inside, and the movement you are about to do. Visualize lifting only from this area.

2

Take a deep breath in and breathe it out slowly. Breathe in again and this time, as you breathe out draw your pelvis toward your chest, pulling your tummy in, not pushing it outward. The movement here is very small and if you have never done any abdominal work, it will be tiny. Don't throw your legs toward your head or use your arms. This only causes a swinging momentum, which takes the emphasis away from your abdomen. It can take a long time to feel these muscles working, or even to feel that they are there at all. They are, and they will be improving if you make the effort to work them regularly.

As you breathe in, slowly lower back to the start position, keeping slight tension in the muscles all the time.

Work the stated number of repetitions and sets.

LOWER ABDOMEN RAISES STRETCH

1

Breathe normally throughout.

Lying with your lower back firmly pressed into the ground, place your arms over your head and relax your upper body.

Bending your knees, place your feet flat on the ground and hip width apart.

2

Reach out with both arms over your head, and feel the stretch from the tummy area continuing up along the trunk of the body and up into the arms, while keeping the lower back in contact with the ground.

Hold the stretch for 8-10 seconds when you warm up, for 20-30 seconds as part of your cool down, then relax.

Fitness for the day
Walk 15 mins

This week's exercise is the lower abdomen raise; read over the coaching points and study the photographs. Note how relaxed the neck, shoulders and arms should be. This is important – you must focus all your attention and effort on your lower abdomen. Take your time, and you will feel that you are doing it properly.

Exercise 1: Wall press 8–10 reps, 2 sets
Exercise 2: Leg extension 6–8 reps, 2 sets
Exercise 3: Lower abdomen raise 4–6 reps, 1 set

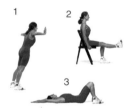

FEELING SCALE FOR EXERCISE

20 MAXIMUM EXERTION

19 EXTRA HARD

17 VERY HARD

16 HARDER

15 HARD

12 LIGHT

10 VERY LIGHT

Food for the day

Breakfast

Snack

Lunch

Snack

Evening meal
Homemade pizza – sounds like a lot of work, but when you've tasted it, you will never want a takeaway again

Light snack

★ Goal for the week
Think back to your long-term goal and pick something along the way.

★ Fitness goal
Did you make all of last week's? If not, repeat one now.

Mood for the day
Mood at the start of the day
Mood at the end of the day

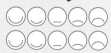

Food tips
Avoid multipacks. Why torture yourself?

Motivation tips
You can say no. Practise in front of the mirror, get used to it.

Fitness for the day
Walk 10 mins

You must be feeling better from this 10-minute interlude in your day, think about how the walk makes you feel. Are you full of energy and stimulated after it? Think about it and note down in the diary how good you feel after it. Walk tall, keeping your ribcage high and abdominals pulled in. Don't forget to breathe normally throughout.

★ Food goal
How's the caffeine intake? Might that be a goal?

FEELING SCALE FOR EXERCISE

20
MAXIMUM EXERTION

19
EXTRA HARD

17
VERY HARD

16
HARDER

15
HARD

12
LIGHT

10
VERY LIGHT

Food for the day

Breakfast

Snack

Lunch
Fresh fruit or juice

Snack

Evening meal

Light snack

★ Goal for the week
Has this week started well?

Mood for the day

Mood at the start of the day

Mood at the end of the day

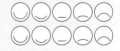

Fitness tips
Keep your walks varied.

Motivation tips
Be honest with yourself.

WEEK THREE DAY THREE

Fitness for the day
Walk 10 mins

You should be feeling more comfortable with the wall press now that you are into your third week. Ask yourself if you can feel it working your chest and shoulders. Could you do more? Do you need to do them slower? Enjoy the sensation of your body working and improving.

Exercise 1: Wall press 8–10 reps, 2 sets
Exercise 2: Leg extension 6–8 reps, 2 sets
Exercise 3: Lower abdomen raise 4–6 reps, 2 sets

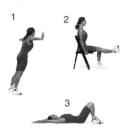

FEELING SCALE FOR EXERCISE

20 MAXIMUM EXERTION

19 EXTRA HARD

17 VERY HARD

16 HARDER

15 HARD

12 LIGHT

10 VERY LIGHT

Food for the day

Breakfast

Snack

Lunch
An enormous mixed salad, dressed with the juice of a lemon and a few twists of freshly milled pepper

Snack

Evening meal

Light snack

★ Goal for the week
Don't lose sight of this – daily goals are important, but this is vital.

★ Fitness goal
If you can't decide, see how many fights of stairs you can make now?

Mood for the day
Mood at the start of the day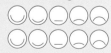
Mood at the end of the day

Food tips
Cook something new today. It will make life more interesing.

Motivation tips
What is most important – gradual, continual weight loss or a quick fix?

Fitness for the day
Walk 10 mins

Make a conscious effort to relax your shoulders as you walk – it's amazing just how tense they can get when you are concentrating on something else. Think about your hands too; try to avoid clenching your fists. You will enjoy it all far more if you relax. Relaxing also makes your workouts a little easier and you will be able to work for longer.
Check your posture constantly.

★ Food goal
Have you cooked a new recipe this week? How about that for today's goal?

FEELING SCALE FOR EXERCISE

20
MAXIMUM EXERTION

19
EXTRA HARD

17
VERY HARD

16
HARDER

15
HARD

12
LIGHT

10
VERY LIGHT

Food for the day

Breakfast

Snack

Lunch

Snack

Evening meal
Risotto – throw in any bits you have left – vegetables, tuna, olives – but cut back on the oil

Light snack

★ Goal for the week
Are you going to make it?

Mood for the day
Mood at the start of the day
Mood at the end of the day

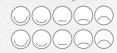

Fitness tips
Check out the local leisure centre. If something sounds interesting, persuade a friend to come too.

Motivation tips
Keep at it – exercise will soon feel part of your life.

Fitness for the day
Walk 10 mins

Keep your back upright, and try to be aware of how tall you are walking. Relax your face and try smiling (not too much – people will think you are strange!). Occasionally, throughout your walk, or when you are stretching, spend some time moving and rolling your shoulders; this will help to keep you loose and relaxed.

★ **Fitness goal**

If you can't decide, see if you can run to the bus stop or station. Warm up first.

FEELING SCALE FOR EXERCISE

20 MAXIMUM EXERTION

19 EXTRA HARD

17 VERY HARD

16 HARDER

15 HARD

12 LIGHT

10 VERY LIGHT

Food for the day

Breakfast

Toasted brown bread with sugar-free jam, no butter or margarine

Snack

Lunch

Snack

Evening meal

Light snack

★ **Goal for the week**
Still on course?

Mood for the day

Mood at the start of the day

Mood at the end of the day

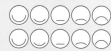

Food tips
Fresh is best – fruit, vegetables, fish.

Motivation tips
You have all the willpower in the world. Use it!

Fitness for the day
Walk 10 mins

Don't get complacent. Keep up a good pace – remember you should be working within the 15–16–17 range to encourage your body to use more energy, to burn fuel and reduce body fat. You need to breathe harder than when you're relaxing, but not so hard as to become breathless. Breathlessness means shortage of oxygen, so slow down a little.

★ **Food goal**
How about one less cup of tea or coffee?

FEELING SCALE FOR EXERCISE

20
MAXIMUM EXERTION

19
EXTRA HARD

17
VERY HARD

16
HARDER

15
HARD

12
LIGHT

10
VERY LIGHT

Food for the day

Breakfast

Snack

Lunch

Snack

Evening meal

Light snack

Grilled tomatoes on toast, topped with chopped fresh basil

★ **Goal for the week**
Are you still going to make it?

Mood for the day

Mood at the start of the day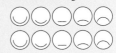
Mood at the end of the day

Fitness tips
Each step, each rep, each set brings you nearer your goal.

Motivation tips
Be prepared for crises, and don't worry about them.

WEEK THREE DAY SEVEN

Fitness for the day
Walk 10 mins

Power up those arms, drive them forward from your elbows and press them backward through your elbows. As you press forward, feel the movement into your forearm rather than out through your hand. Make your walk a good strong one, one that you know you have worked hard at, but don't jeopardize your technique. Walk with style and good posture.

Well done. You've spent nearly a month of doing something for you, that's going to last for the rest of your life.

★ Fitness goal
Hassle the local sports centre about creche facilities - it will all help you and others in the future.

FEELING SCALE FOR EXERCISE

20 MAXIMUM EXERTION

19 EXTRA HARD

17 VERY HARD

16 HARDER

15 HARD

12 LIGHT

10 VERY LIGHT

Food for the day
Breakfast

Snack

Lunch
Baked pasta shells in tomato, onion and low-fat yogurt sauce, with lots of fresh herbs

Snack

Evening meal

Light snack

★ Goal for the week
Did you make it – well done you!

Mood for the day
Mood at the start of the day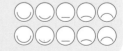
Mood at the end of the day

Food tips
A level spoonful is half as much as a rounded one. Be conscious of what you are eating, especially sugars.

Motivation tips
Being realistic works. You know it does. Stick at it.

WEEK FOUR INTRODUCTION

Excellent, one whole month, four whole weeks, 28 whole days – doesn't that sound good? I bet you're feeling good, not just for getting this far, but more for how it has made you feel and the benefits you have derived from taking the first step on your ladder to a fuller life, with plenty of energy and minimal stress. Make a conscious effort to smile a lot this week to celebrate achieving so much in your first step.

This week you are focusing on a full 10 minutes' daily walking, to be sure that it is now firmly part of your routine. It really does take a minimum of four weeks to make a new habit habitual (and sometimes longer to be rid of an unhealthy one). Stay with it, you're doing brilliantly.

Get the family out walking with you – they need the fresh air and exercise too, so start setting them up with good new habits to match your own. You will all benefit from this effort. If you've got children, make it a game: who can walk the fastest? pump their arms the highest? reach the tree first? Have some fun.

Keep your food diary and your mood faces filled in – at the end of this week you have your first month's assessment (see pp. 71–2). I'm sure you already have seen certain patterns forming in your eating and drinking habits, which is why it is so important that you are honest with yourself. This book is for you: only you can see where your strengths and weaknesses lie. Only by looking back over the weeks can you see how many days you walked and how many days you did the exercises.

As the weeks progress, so will your ability to take charge of yourself. This will make your goals that much easier to obtain. And when you achieve your goals, you open the door to opportunities that only a few short weeks ago you might have considered beyond your wildest dreams.

This week you are working the back of your arms. This neglected area shows fat deposits quickly. This exercise, however, is very effective and it will not take long to show results if you do it regularly. At the same time, it's important to work the front of your arms, which we'll get to in a couple of weeks (see pp. 94–5). You will be amazed how much shape you can give your arms, and how much you will appreciate having some strength in them. Strength here takes the stress off many of the major muscles of your upper body – your shoulders, back and chest.

TRICEP EXTENSION

You can do this exercise standing or sitting, although I usually sit as the body tends to be more stable when you are seated and your back is under less pressure. It also means you can focus on your arms, without worrying about how you are standing.

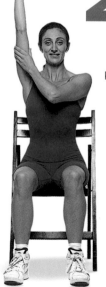

1
Warm up and stretch, using movements that mobilize your shoulders and arms.

Sit with your knees and feet hip width apart and your feet flat on the floor. Keep your back straight, ribcage lifted and lower and upper abdominal muscles pulled in. Relax your shoulders.

Extend your right arm over your head. Place your left hand on the underside of your right arm for added support but check that you don't alter your posture.

Keeping your neck and shoulders relaxed, and your head in line with your spine, breathe in as you bend your right arm at the elbow and reach down with your hand behind your neck toward the centre of your shoulder blades.

2
Try to keep your elbow pointing upward.

Breathe out as you extend your right hand toward the sky. Stop slightly short of full extension, so that you don't lock your elbow.

Keep a little tension in the muscle, as you start the next repetition. Use the air as a resistance – imagine you are pushing through mud or treacle – as you work the arm both up and down and don't worry about how far down your back you get your hand. Also keep your head upright (it's very easy to let it fall forward).

Complete a set with your right arm, then repeat using your left arm. Work the stated number of reps and sets with each arm.

TRICEP STRETCH

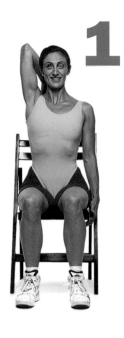

1

Sit on a chair or on the floor with your back straight, ribcage lifted and tummy pulled in. Relax your shoulders and keep your head in line with your spine.

Extend your right arm above your head, bending it at the elbow and letting your hand fall toward the back of your neck.

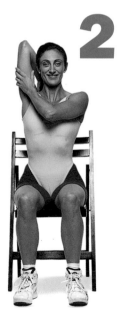

2

Gently use your left hand to press and firmly hold the back of your extended right arm. Keep your elbow pointing upward, easing the arm into the stretch. Press toward the back of your body.

You should feel a good stretch in the back of your arm, from your shoulder to your elbow. Be sure to keep your head upright and shoulders relaxed. Hold this position and feel the tension ease away.

Hold the stretch for 8–10 seconds when you warm up, for 20–30 seconds as part of your cool down, then relax.

Repeat with your left arm.

Fitness for the day
Walk 10 mins

Back to your upper body for this week's new exercise, the triceps (in other words, the backs of your arms) extension. This is the area that can look so bad when the sun shines and you want to wear a sleeveless vest. It will not take long before you start to notice a difference in the tone of the muscles here, but if you are carrying a lot of body fat, a fair proportion may be lodged here, so work on reducing your fat and sugar intake too, and keep up the vigorous walking for best results.

Exercise 1: Wall press
10–12 reps, 2 sets
Exercise 2: Leg extension
8–10 reps, 2 sets
Exercise 3: Lower abdomen raise 6–8 reps, 2 sets
Exercise 4: Tricep extension
4–6 reps, 1 set

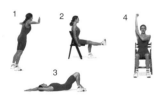

FEELING SCALE FOR EXERCISE

20 MAXIMUM EXERTION

19 EXTRA HARD

17 VERY HARD

16 HARDER

15 HARD

12 LIGHT

10 VERY LIGHT

Food for the day

Breakfast

Home-made muffins – be adventurous, try blueberry or lemon flavour

Snack

Lunch

Snack

Evening meal

Light snack

★ Goal for the week

Choose one, write it down, and stick to it!

★ Food goal

Keep at it – have you abandoned one 'poor' food yet?

Mood for the day

Mood at the start of the day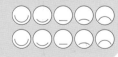

Mood at the end of the day

Fitness tips

Take time to look around you as you walk. Enjoy your surroundings.

Motivation tips

You are not alone in being unhappy in life – many people are. But there's a difference – you can change your life.

WEEK FOUR DAY TWO

Fitness for the day
Walk 10 mins

You should be feeling that you can fit 10 minutes into your day quite nicely: it really does not take long to build a good habit into your routine. Your body will appreciate what you are doing for it, and all the while you are making yourself feel good too. Keep walking at a pace that encourages you to breathe slightly more heavily, feel your body temperature start to rise, take in that fresh air and energize your body.

★ Fitness goal

How about borrowing the neighbour's dog and taking it for a run in the park?

FEELING SCALE FOR EXERCISE

20
MAXIMUM EXERTION

19
EXTRA HARD

17
VERY HARD

16
HARDER

15
HARD

12
LIGHT

10
VERY LIGHT

Food for the day

Breakfast

Snack

Lunch

Granary bread sandwich filled with cottage cheese and pineapple

Snack

Evening meal

Light snack

★ Goal for the week

How about wanting to feel really good?

Food tips

Take herb teas and lemons with you when you visit friends – you don't have to have tea or coffee simply because they do.

Mood for the day

Mood at the start of the day

Mood at the end of the day

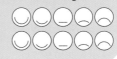

Motivation tips

Share your feelings – the sooner you confront the demons, the better.

Fitness for the day
Walk 10 mins

Make a conscious effort to focus your mind on the muscles you are working. It really does take time to feel these exercises properly, to isolate those muscles that you are working now. Keep reading and studying the photographs until you feel confident that you are working the right muscles, and that your posture is correct and supporting and helping your body where necessary.

Exercise 1: Wall press
10–12 reps, 2 sets
Exercise 2: Leg extension
8–10 reps, 2 sets
Exercise 3: Lower abdomen
raise 6–8 rep,s 2 sets
Exercise 4: Tricep extension
4–6 reps, 2 sets

FEELING SCALE FOR EXERCISE

20 MAXIMUM EXERTION

19 EXTRA HARD

17 VERY HARD

16 HARDER

15 HARD

12 LIGHT

10 VERY LIGHT

Food for the day

Breakfast

Snack

Lunch
Couscous, with fresh raw chopped vegetables and lemon juice dressing – delicious!

Snack

Evening meal

Light snack

★ Goal for the week
How's it going?

Mood for the day

Mood at the start of the day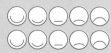

Mood at the end of the day

★ Food goal
You know your weaknesses – what is it to be?

Fitness tips
Every step you take, you are burning fat.

Motivation tips
Praise yourself every day for what you have achieved – you are doing marvellously.

Fitness for the day
Walk 10 mins

Keep your walk energetic, challenge your body to walk faster. If you find a slight hill, make the effort to feel your buttocks working too, pump those arms to help you get there. Keep your back straight and upper and lower abdominals pulled in, lift your ribcage, expand your chest and take in huge lungs full of air. Stoke up the fuel burners and get those muscles working.

★ Fitness goal
Climbed any stairs lately?

FEELING SCALE FOR EXERCISE

20
MAXIMUM EXERTION

19
EXTRA HARD

17
VERY HARD

16
HARDER

15
HARD

12
LIGHT

10
VERY LIGHT

Food for the day

Breakfast

Snack

Lemon scones (add the juice and rind to the mix), sprinkle with poppy seeds the minute they come out of the oven

Lunch

Snack

Evening meal

Light snack

★ Goal for the week
Keep it up!

Mood for the day

Mood at the start of the day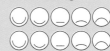

Mood at the end of the day

Food tips
Use a non-stick frying pan and fry fat free – you will be amazed at the taste of the food, not the oil!

Motivation tips
You can have anything you want if you want it enough.

Fitness for the day
Walk 10 mins

Each day you are fitter, more energized, more positive, and better able to deal with what the day has to offer. While you are walking, think about what this walk means to you. Try walking a little further today, making your legs stretch out. Feel them getting firmer as you make a conscious effort to walk with purpose.

★ Food goal
Enjoy every mouthful – really notice what you are eating.

FEELING SCALE FOR EXERCISE

20 MAXIMUM EXERTION

19 EXTRA HARD

17 VERY HARD

16 HARDER

15 HARD

12 LIGHT

10 VERY LIGHT

Food for the day
Breakfast
Egg white omelette filled with leftover vegetables – great when you have time for something hot

Snack

Lunch

Snack

Evening meal

Light snack

★ Goal for the week
How's it going – this is nearly the end of the first month.

Mood for the day
Mood at the start of the day
Mood at the end of the day

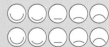

Fitness tips
Pump your arms, get your body moving, kick start that metabolism.

Motivation tips
You have already taken the biggest step; now just stick with it.

Fitness for the day
Walk 10 mins

Take a good look in the mirror before you go out for your walk – you will see how much better you look for making the effort to do something for you and your body every day. Smile at yourself, you have every right to feel good. Now get out there and walk, keep that head high, your shoulders relaxed, ribcage lifted and abdominals pulled in.

★ Fitness goal

There are scores to choose from, but you are the only person who counts. What do you need to do?

FEELING SCALE FOR EXERCISE

20
MAXIMUM EXERTION

19
EXTRA HARD

17
VERY HARD

16
HARDER

15
HARD

12
LIGHT

10
VERY LIGHT

Food for the day
Breakfast

Snack

Lunch

Mixed bean salad, with an orange juice dressing, sprinkled with fresh parsley – you won't know how good it is until you try it!

Snack

Evening meal

Light snack

★ Goal for the week
Are you going to make it?

Mood for the day

Mood at the start of the day

Mood at the end of the day

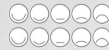

Food tips
Use bran or chickpea flour to thicken soups and stews.

Motivation tips
Old habits do die hard, but once you've established some new ones, the old ones fade away.

Fitness for the day

Walk 10 mins

One whole month, that's brilliant! Today is a big day, it's assessment day and measuring day. Use a tape measure or your clothes to see how well you have done. Remember that this change is going to be gradual, without too much pressure on your time and to keep a sense of balance in your life.

Think about what you have learned about yourself and your body and how you can use this as you go into the second month. Well done and good luck!

★ Food goal

Don't take any notice of what others may think of your goals. Do what is right for you.

FEELING SCALE FOR EXERCISE

20
MAXIMUM
EXERTION

19
EXTRA
HARD

17
VERY
HARD

16
HARDER

15
HARD

12
LIGHT

10
VERY
LIGHT

Food for the day

Breakfast

Snack

Lunch

Snack

Crudités with hot and spicy salsa dip

Evening meal

Light snack

★ Goal for the week

Did you make it – well done you!

Mood for the day

Mood at the
start of the day

Mood at the end
of the day

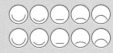

Fitness tips

Don't forsake control or technique to do another repetition. Do fewer with good technique.

Motivation tips

Don't intend it. Do it!

ASSESSMENT

You can tell how well you are doing with the programme by simply keeping a pair of trousers or a skirt and trying it on once a month to see how much better it fits you. Since *First Steps to Fitness* is about more than your waistline, however, this monthly assessment will help you to see what is happening in all areas of your life.

Fitness and food assessment

At the end of each week add up how many times you reached your goal and note it on the grid. Did you achieve more goals in week four than week one? Or did you perhaps start off with some of your goals a little too easy? Are you finding it easier on the whole to reach fitness targets than food one – check back and see.

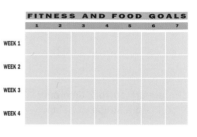

How did you feel after exercise? Are you noticing improvements? Do you feel less tired, better able to cope? And what about food? Was there a particularly bad week and did it coincide with stress in another area of your life? Or did you perhaps eat late a few days, which upset your resolve? Think about why you eats as well as what you eat, to see if you are using food for comfort or other emotional reasons.

6–7 goals per week

This is excellent, but are you perhaps making them a bit easy? If you are consistently scoring 6–7, you are obviously determined and may be fitter and have more willpower than you thought. Try upping the pace a little, and make things a bit more difficult.

4–5 goals per week

Excellent. You are making an effort, have obviously chosen realistic goals that you can achieve with time and practice. Try not to fall below this level and aim for a week or two at 6 or 7 next month.

3 goals per week

Good. Don't be discouraged, this is a good start. You have acknowledged you need to change and you have started to do something about it. Well done. Aim for a couple of 4s or 5s next month – remember this is all about gradually changing.

1–2 goals per week

Keep trying. Don't be beaten. You have made a good start and next month you will achieve more. If you are consistently not reaching fitness goals, are you making them a bit too difficult? Don't rush it, you have the rest of your life. Get your mind and body into gear and away you go.

ASSESSMENT

Feeling scale assessment

Add up the entries on your feeling scales and note them on the grid. Were you gradually able to work a bit harder as the month progressed, or did you constantly feel out of breath. Aim to work at 15–16–17 all the time; 10 is too low and 20 is dangerous. Could you have pumped harder with your arms? Could you have resisted more with the exercises? Think about it as you exercise and note how you feel.

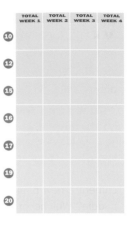

Mood scale assessment

Fill in the mood grids for the beginning and end of each day. Does your mood tend to improve over the course of the day or get worse? Do you constantly wake up feeling bad? Are you having too many late nights? Too many late meals, perhaps with alcohol? If you do find your mood worsening over the day, think about what is happening. And check your food diary and see if there are any foods that trigger bad moods. Does your daily walk improve your mood?

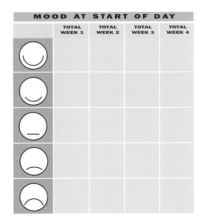

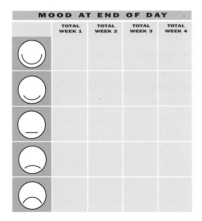

WEEK FIVE INTRODUCTION

Week five and into the second month already. Fantastic! I trust you are feeling good and enjoying yourself. Did the end-of-month assessment convince you how well you are doing?

Having a good balance in life is important for your well-being. The diary format of this book will enable you to watch your progress and allow you to work on specific areas in your life that you might want to change, and at the same time introduce you into exercise to maintain and improve on what you have already.

You should now feel comfortable about filling in the food diary honestly. After last week's assessment, you should have sorted out your goals for this next step, these next four weeks. Are you continuing with your previous goal, to cement a new habit firmly into your life, or rid yourself for good of a real baddie? Whichever it is, good for you – it takes a lot of effort but it will be all worth it, just wait and see. Keep your goals simple and they will slowly materialize.

You are already doing great things – walking 10 minutes a day (which over this week we will increase to 15 minutes). Keep the pace up. Focus on your technique, be sure to roll through your feet and to squeeze deep into the muscles in your buttocks. Keep your arms up and pumping, make your heart beat harder and breathe in deeper, fill your body with oxygen.

You should by now be feeling very confident with the first three exercises, but take your time with the repetitions and flick back to the photographs and coaching points to make sure that your technique is correct. You are also into your second week of triceps extensions so check over the coaching points and focus on using the correct muscles.

And now for week five and shoulder shrugs. These are for your upper back and shoulders. A weakness here tends to let you pull your shoulders forward, and they start to round (this is particularly noticeable in people who sit at a desk all day). Think of the strain you put on your upper back when you carry shopping or pick up the children. Your body can only cope with so much stress before something has to give – your neck aches, your shoulders are tense, your lower back aches, and so on.

SHOULDER SHRUG

You can do this exercise standing or sitting, but I prefer to sit for stability. Breathe normally throughout.

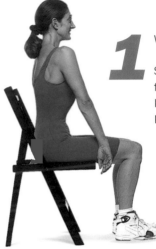

1 Warm up and stretch.

Sit with your knees and feet hip width apart, and your feet flat on the floor. Keep your back straight, ribcage lifted and tummy pulled in. Relax your shoulders and keep your head in line with your spine. Look forward.

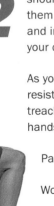

2 Relax your arms by your sides. Slowly lift your shoulders forward and then upward and slowly roll them backward and down, keeping your head upright and in line with your spine. Don't be tempted to lower your chin.

As you rotate your shoulders, do so slowly and try to resist the movement, as if you were making it in treacle or mud. Keep your arms close to your body and hands down by your sides.

Pause when you reach the start position and repeat.

Work the stated number of repetitions and sets.

SHOULDER STRETCH

Breathe normally throughout.

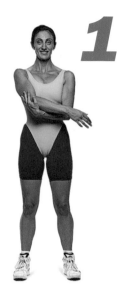

Stand with your knees and feet hip width apart, and your feet flat on. the floor. Keep your back straight, ribcage lifted and tummy pulled in. Relax your shoulders and keep your head in line with your spine. Look forward.

Relax shoulders, and with one hand take hold of the front of your other arm between the shoulder and the elbow.

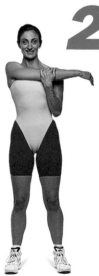

With the active arm, gently pull the other arm across your chest, relaxing your upper back and allowing your shoulder blades to separate as you do so. Keep your tummy pulled in and make sure that your head is in line with your spine.

Your arms will probably be somewhere between chest and shoulder height, but adjust your position according to where you can feel the stretch best.

Hold the stretch for 8–10 seconds when you warm up, for 20–30 seconds as part of your cool down, then relax.

Repeat with the other arm.

Fitness for the day
Walk 10 mins

We're staying with the upper body this week with an exercise for your back. Take time out to mobilize your shoulders, then your neck before you start, then do the exercise slowly, studying the coaching points and photographs. Feel the muscles working and focus on keeping the rest of your body stable.

Exercise 1: Wall press 12–14 reps, 2 sets
Exercise 2: Leg extension 10–12 reps, 2 sets
Exercise 3: Lower abdomen raise 8–10 reps, 2 sets
Exercise 4: Tricep extension 6–8 reps, 2 sets
Exercise 5: Shoulder shrug 4–6 reps, 1 set

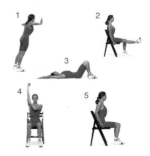

FEELING SCALE FOR EXERCISE

20 MAXIMUM EXERTION

19 EXTRA HARD

17 VERY HARD

16 HARDER

15 HARD

12 LIGHT

10 VERY LIGHT

Food for the day

Breakfast

Snack

Lunch

Snack

Evening meal
Soya chilli with rice

Light snack

★ Goal for the week
Why not give yourself a challenge this week?

★ Fitness goal
Only you know what to choose.

Mood for the day

Mood at the start of the day
Mood at the end of the day

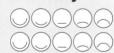

Food tips
Alter the balance of your plate – the largest helping should be carbohydrate (rice, pasta, potatoes), next a portion of vegetables or salad, then a modest portion of meat, fish or other protein.

Motivation tips
Keep it simple, one step at a time.

Fitness for the day

Walk 10–11 mins

Increase your walk by a minute today, and make a conscious effort to take big strides and really use your arms to resist the air around them. Into your second month, smile deeply at yourself and praise your efforts for continuing and maintaining this level of intensity. You know how much of an effort you made. If you honestly could have done more, make that your fitness goal for tomorrow. If you know you made a good effort, note in the diary how this made you feel.

★ Food goal

You know what you need to do. Write it down here and now.

FEELING SCALE FOR EXERCISE

20 MAXIMUM EXERTION

19 EXTRA HARD

17 VERY HARD

16 HARDER

15 HARD

12 LIGHT

10 VERY LIGHT

Food for the day

Breakfast

Snack

Lunch

Jacket potato loaded with goodies – tuna, prawns, salad, raw vegetables, hot or cold

Snack

Evening meal

Light snack

★ Goal for the week

Have you started how you mean to go on?

Mood for the day

Mood at the start of the day

Mood at the end of the day

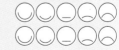

Fitness tips

When the going gets tough, count the reps down rather than up.

Motivation tips

You are not just doing this for you. Think about your children and do it for them too.

77

WEEK FIVE DAY THREE

Fitness for the day
Walk 11 mins

Aim to reach the maximum reps and sets for the day. Do each repetition slowly and try to focus on the muscles you are using and how they seem to be taking to the exercise. Does it feel right? Is it comfortable? Is your posture correct when you do the exercises? Keep looking at the photographs and reading the coaching points. Perhaps you need to work a bit slower? Could you do more repetitions? Note down how you felt in the diary.

Exercise 1: Wall press 12–14 reps, 2 sets
Exercise 2: Leg extension 10–12 reps, 2 sets
Exercise 3: Lower abdominal raise 8–10 reps, 2 sets
Exercise 4: Tricep extension 6–8 reps, 2 sets
Exercise 5: Shoulder shrug 4–6 reps, 2 sets

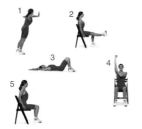

FEELING SCALE FOR EXERCISE

20 MAXIMUM EXERTION

19 EXTRA HARD

17 VERY HARD

16 HARDER

15 HARD

12 LIGHT

10 VERY LIGHT

Food for the day

Breakfast

A fresh juice – quick, simple, light on the stomach and delicious

Snack

Lunch

Snack

Evening meal

Light snack

★ Goal for the week
How's it going?

★ Fitness goal
It is boring to climb stairs, but such good exercise. Keep trying with this.

Mood for the day

Mood at the start of the day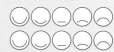
Mood at the end of the day

Food tips
Make your own low-fat or fat-free salad dressings and take them with you when you eat out.

Motivation tips
You can't make others happy by ignoring your own needs.

78

Fitness for the day
Walk 11–12 mins

Yes, another whole minute, go for it and enjoy the extra time to yourself. Don't shuffle along, but walk those legs, pick your feet up and stride out. Get some oxygen inside you, start to feel your body come to life – feeling good, knowing that you are building a healthier body to fend off illness and depression is what it's all about.

★ Food goal
Do you eat when you are bored? Make a conscious effort to conquer boredom.

FEELING SCALE FOR EXERCISE

20
MAXIMUM EXERTION

19
EXTRA HARD

17
VERY HARD

16
HARDER

15
HARD

12
LIGHT

10
VERY LIGHT

Food for the day
Breakfast

Snack

Lunch

Snack

Chick pea delight. Soak and cook the peas, then mould into 'cakes'; bake until crunchy

Evening meal

Light snack

★ Goal for the week
Keep it up!

Mood for the day
Mood at the start of the day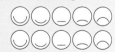
Mood at the end of the day

Fitness tips
The harder you exercise the more fat you will burn.

Motivation tips
Remember the three Ds – desire, drive, dedication.

Fitness for the day
Walk 12 mins

Enjoy your walk, put a smile on your face and feel the energy coursing through your body, each and every day. As you step out, you are gradually building your fitness level, reminding your body that it does work, that it can function on all cylinders, even after years of neglect, given the opportunity.

★ Fitness goal
Remember that you are building toward a better life – too little at this stage is probably better than too much. Be realistic.

FEELING SCALE FOR EXERCISE

20 MAXIMUM EXERTION

19 EXTRA HARD

17 VERY HARD

16 HARDER

15 HARD

12 LIGHT

10 VERY LIGHT

Food for the day

Breakfast

Pick up an Asian habit and try leftover rice, delicious with chopped fresh fruit

Snack

Lunch

Snack

Evening meal

Light snack

★ Goal for the week
How are you doing?

Mood for the day

Mood at the start of the day

Mood at the end of the day

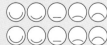

Food tips
Use low-fat natural yogurt to thicken soups and casseroles.

Motivation tips
Believe in yourself. You can do it.

Fitness for the day

Walk 12–13 mins

How is your posture? Are you still consciously making an effort to keep it all upright and tucked in? Are you standing and walking tall, lifting your ribcage, breathing easily? Get your shoulders back and down, relax and walk with a sense of purpose.

★ Food goal

Food is a family battle ground. Don't succumb.

FEELING SCALE FOR EXERCISE

20
MAXIMUM EXERTION

19
EXTRA HARD

17
VERY HARD

16
HARDER

15
HARD

12
LIGHT

10
VERY LIGHT

Food for the day

Breakfast

Snack

As much fresh fruit as you can eat

Lunch

Snack

Evening meal

Light snack

★ Goal for the week

You're nearly there? How do you feel?

Mood for the day

Mood at the start of the day

Mood at the end of the day

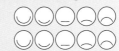

Fitness tips

If your energy levels are low, listen to your body. You can make up tomorrow.

Motivation tips

You can learn to say no.

Fitness for the day
Walk 13–15 mins

Excellent! Do you realize that you are halfway to your goal of 30 minutes. You have done brilliantly. Take time to feel your body's movements, enjoy the feeling of freedom that comes with moving with ease. Breathe more deeply and exhale slowly, appreciating the air you are taking in. Think about what all that oxygen is doing – it's energizing you, making you feel good. Your whole appearance will take on a newer and fresher look. Enjoy your brisk walk!

★ Fitness goal
You now know that the key word is realistic, don't you?

FEELING SCALE FOR EXERCISE

20
MAXIMUM
EXERTION

19
EXTRA
HARD

17
VERY
HARD

16
HARDER

15
HARD

12
LIGHT

10
VERY
LIGHT

Food for the day

Breakfast

Snack

Lunch

Potato skins with broccoli and tofu filling

Snack

Evening meal

Light snack

★ Goal for the week
Did you make it?

Mood for the day

Mood at the start of the day

Mood at the end of the day

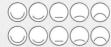

Food tips
Use fresh lemon, lime and orange in your salad dressings.

Motivation tips
Saying no does not reflect badly on the person offering.

WEEK SIX *INTRODUCTION*

This is a major marker in your diary, not only are you halfway into your walking programme, you are also halfway through your 12-week programme and into your sixth exercise. You definitely deserve a pat on the back. Perhaps you feel like celebrating or maybe you want to get through the whole 12 weeks before you plan anything? Celebrating, of course, does not mean blowing everything you have worked so hard to achieve so far. This programme is not about deprivation and binges; it's about making changes slowly, educating your body and your mind to want better things. There are all sorts of celebrations: perhaps you should make one your goal – a new (smaller) suit, an exercise outfit, a juicer, a trip to the theatre or a concert or sporting event, the list is endless.

Moderation is the key word for this week. You're going to be doing a straight 15 minutes walk each day so that when you up the time next week, your body will be able to cope without too much stress or effort. Do you look forward to this time? Are you enjoying your walks? Do you like the feeling as you return from your walk? Are you energized? Full of enthusiasm? Exercise affects people in so many different ways. Continue to monitor your moods. Are you affected more by your food than your walk or do both play an equal part? Think about how you feel after you have eaten? Did it fill you up? Did it make you tired? Or buzzing full of energy?

This week you start a split routine, so that you can incorporate all the exercises without rushing or making a single session too time consuming. This way of working also prevents you from feeling exhausted from the added workload. This week's new exercise is the calf raise for the muscles at the back of the lower leg, which connect your heel to your foot, and then run up into the back of your knee. A lot of people have quite strong calves, and you may only need to tone yours – high repetitions will do this. But if you have weaker or less developed muscles here, you need to build up the reps and eventually increase the resistance for strength and definition.

To strengthen the small muscle on the front of the calf that runs midway up from the bone toward your knee, you need to do toe taps. Raise your toes up toward your shin, keeping your heel in contact with the floor throughout. If you drive a manual car, then you should have pretty good strength and development in the front of your shin, since the movement of clutch and accelerator control is like toe tapping. If you have an automatic car, this muscle will be better developed in one leg than the other. Have a look; if they are uneven, work on the weaker one, gradually building up the repetitions. Constantly wearing high-heeled shoes has a gradual shortening effect on the calf muscle, which could lead to real problems when you are older. Help yourself by doing lots of stretching in this area. And, if you can, stop wearing high heels, or keep them for one-off occasions rather than everyday wear.

CALF RAISE

Calf raises can also be done standing, which allows you to use your whole body weight as a resistance to increase the workload on your muscles. Use this as a progression: when you feel you are working as hard as you can sitting, do them standing.

You can increase the resistance by placing a large book on your thighs,: put your hands firmly on top of the book to cover both your thighs, and resist on both the up and down movements. This exercise can also be performed with your toes turned slightly outward and heels closer together to emphasize the outer part of your calf muscle; similarly turning your toes inward emphasizes the inner part of the muscle.

Breathe normally throughout.

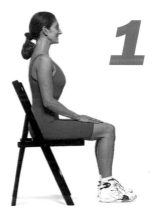

1

If you are doing this exercise straight after your walk, your muscles should be warm already. If not, warm up and stretch.

Sit with your feet and knees hip width apart and your feet flat on the floor. Keep your back straight, ribcage lifted and tummy pulled in. Relax your shoulders and keep your head in line with your spine.

Slide your feet slightly back under the chair so that your toes are more in line with your knees.

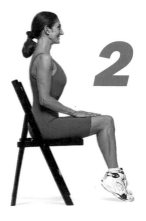

2

Resisting the floor, slowly raise up on to the balls of your feet, pause and squeeze into the muscle.

Resist the air as you slowly lower your heels back down to the floor; imagine you are making the movement through mud or treacle. Concentrate on the movement and try to ensure that your ankles don't roll out to the side.

Work the stated numbers of repetitions and sets.

CALF STRETCH

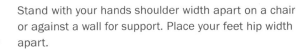

1 Stand with your hands shoulder width apart on a chair or against a wall for support. Place your feet hip width apart.

Check that your back is straight, ribcage lifted, lower and upper abdominals pulled in, shoulders relaxed and head in line with your spine.

2 Bending your left knee slightly, take a large step backward with your right foot. As you do so, check that your feet are still hip width apart and facing forward. Look to see where your feet are positioned. Your supporting knee should be midway between your shoelaces and your toes.

Press the heel of your right foot firmly down, keeping your back straight and tummy pulled in . Feel the stretch from the back of your knee, down to your heel. If you can't feel it, slide your foot back a fraction, until you feel your calf muscle stretching.

Hold the stretch for 8–10 seconds when you warm up, for 20–30 seconds as part of your cool down, then relax. Repeat with your other leg.

Fitness for the day
Walk 15 mins

You are now on to 3 sets of the wall press, well done. Take your time and ensure good technique throughout all repetitions and all sets. If you miss a couple of sessions, you may have to do fewer repetitions, so make a note to yourself in the diary and gradually build back up again. If you are finding it all too easy, increase the number of repetitions and, if you really feel up to it, the sets. You know your body best, so do what you feel comfortable with.

Exercise 1: Wall press
14–16 reps, 3 sets
Exercise 2: Leg extension
12–14 reps, 2 sets
Exercise 3: Lower abdomen raise 10–12 reps, 2 sets
Exercise 4: Tricep extension 8–10 reps, 2 sets
Exercise 5: Shoulder shrug 6–8 reps, 2 sets

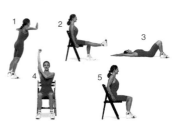

FEELING SCALE FOR EXERCISE

20 MAXIMUM EXERTION

19 EXTRA HARD

17 VERY HARD

16 HARDER

15 HARD

12 LIGHT

10 VERY LIGHT

Food for the day
Breakfast

Stewed rhubarb - add a squeeze of lemon and some grated ginger and really wake your mouth up

Snack

Lunch

Snack

Evening meal

Light snack

★ Goal for the week
Choose yours – and go for it!

★ Food goal
Is there one from last week still needing work?

Mood for the day

Mood at the start of the day

Mood at the end of the day

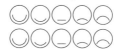

Fitness tips
Your metabolism may take longer than someone else's to kick start – but keep walking and you will start to burn fat.

Motivation tips
To change the way you look, you have to change the way you think.

Fitness for the day
Walk 15 mins

This week, here and now, you are at the halfway point on your first programme, putting you firmly on that first step of the ladder to a fitter, happier and healthier you. How do you feel? Get out and burn some of that excess you have been storing in those fat pouches. Make the effort to pump your arms and work from your shoulders, through to your hands. Use the air as a resistance and get your heart pumping.

★ Fitness goal
A new day, a new goal. What is it to be today?

FEELING SCALE FOR EXERCISE

20 MAXIMUM EXERTION

19 EXTRA HARD

17 VERY HARD

16 HARDER

15 HARD

12 LIGHT

10 VERY LIGHT

Food for the day

Breakfast

Snack

Lunch

Snack

Evening meal
Grilled trout sprinkled with fresh herbs, with rice or new potatoes and a large salad

Light snack

★ Goal of the week
Are you enjoying the challenge?

Mood for the day

Mood at the start of the day

Mood at the end of the day

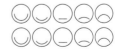

Food tips
Chocolates, biscuits, salted nuts and savoury snacks trigger binges. Don't buy them.

Motivation tips
Liking yourself is the first step toward others liking you.

Fitness for the day
Walk 15 mins

Aim for the maximum sets and reps in all the exercises. Remember that your muscles move in two directions, both of which need to be worked in equal amounts, so resist the movements up slowly and down again slowly. You will find that your body and mind are working better together as your hand–eye co-ordination improves. Well done, stay with it!

Exercise 1: Wall press
14–16 reps, 3 sets
Exercise 2: Leg extension
12–14 reps, 2 sets
Exercise 3: Lower abdomen
raise 10–12 reps, 2 sets
Exercise 4: Tricep extension
8–10 reps, 2 sets
Exercise 5: Shoulder shrug
6–8 reps, 2 sets

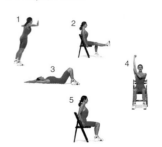

FEELING SCALE FOR EXERCISE

20 MAXIMUM EXERTION

19 EXTRA HARD

17 VERY HARD

16 HARDER

15 HARD

12 LIGHT

10 VERY LIGHT

Food for the day

Breakfast

Snack

Lunch
Rice salad - put in anything and everything you fancy

Snack

Evening meal

Light snack

★ Goal for the week
Keep it up!

★ Food goal
How about trying an exotic new fruit you haven't bought before?

Mood for the day

Mood at the start of the day

Mood at the end of the day

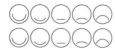

Fitness tips
Buy a kite and get out in the fresh air with it. Breathe in deeply.

Motivation tips
Spend two minutes a day imagining yourself succeeding this time.

Fitness for the day
Walk 15 mins.

How's your posture? Are you feeling more comfortable, aware that you are standing taller, with a straight back? Is your chest lifted? How are those abdominals holding out? If you haven't noticed, why not? Get in touch with your body, take stock of what is happening to your posture, breathe deeply, enjoy the oxygen stimulating and energizing your whole body.

★ Fitness goal
Are you making these too easy or too difficult? Think before you write.

FEELING SCALE FOR EXERCISE

20 MAXIMUM EXERTION

19 EXTRA HARD

17 VERY HARD

16 HARDER

15 HARD

12 LIGHT

10 VERY LIGHT

Food for the day
Breakfast

Snack

Lunch

Snack
Date scones

Evening meal

Light snack

★ Goal for the week
How's it going?

Food tips
At the risk of sounding like your mother – eat your greens, they really are important for all sorts of vitamins and minerals.

Mood for the day
Mood at the start of the day
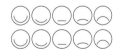

Mood at the end of the day

Motivation tips
Continuity and persistence will get you where you want to be.

Fitness for the day
Walk 15 mins

From here on in, it's up to four sessions of exercises each week. This week's is great for giving some shape and strength to your calves. Make a conscious effort to resist the air on the movement up and down – this makes the exercise far more effective. This is a good exercise to do after your walk, as the calves will be thoroughly warmed through, and receptive to the work you are going to ask them to do.

Exercise 6: Calf raise
4–6 reps, 1 set

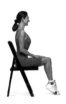

FEELING SCALE FOR EXERCISE

20
MAXIMUM EXERTION
☐

19
EXTRA HARD
☐

17
VERY HARD
☐

16
HARDER
☐

15
HARD
☐

12
LIGHT
☐

10
VERY LIGHT
☐

Food for the day

Breakfast

Snack

Lunch

Snack

Evening meal

Vegetarian shepherds pie. Make it using lentils and spinach in place of the meat, with onions and mushrooms as usual

Light snack

★ Goal for the week
Still on course?

★ Food goal
To treat my tastebuds.

Fitness tips
If you have an exercise bike, pedal while you watch your favourite soap or the evening news – you won't notice the time passing.

Mood for the day

Mood at the start of the day
Mood at the end of the day

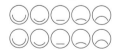

Motivation tips
Don't be trapped by negative thoughts. Start now to think positive.

Fitness for the day
Walk 15 mins

This daily walk is helping you to stay on the right track, through increasing your daily activity level in general. It is also making a new habit, that you can see and feel is doing you good. This should be a spur to cutting down on your fat and sugar intake – you don't need it, nor do you want it. You don't have to steer clear of these things all the time, just more often than not ... and remember it does get easier.

★ Fitness goal
To reward my efforts with a new vest/ teeshirt/ pair of jogging trousers.

FEELING SCALE FOR EXERCISE

20 MAXIMUM EXERTION

19 EXTRA HARD

17 VERY HARD

16 HARDER

15 HARD

12 LIGHT

10 VERY LIGHT

Food for the day
Breakfast
Scrambled tofu – at least give it a try

Snack

Lunch

Snack

Evening meal

Light snack

★ Goal for the week
Keep going, you're nearly there.

Food tips
Folic acid is important in most diets and vital if you are, or thinking about becoming, pregnant. Eat lots of spinach and other green leafy vegetables, citrus fruits and some wholewheat bread (check the label to see if it has been added).

Mood for the day
Mood at the start of the day

Mood at the end of the day

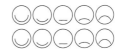

Motivation tips
Don't stop to question your success; get on with it!

Fitness for the day
Walk 15 mins

Well, this week was a full week – how do you feel? You should be proud of what you have achieved, you have done so well, working toward improving your lot, and reaping the rewards of feeling good, enjoying having a little bit more energy, maybe sleeping better. How's your sex life? Do you feel enthused?. Does your partner need to start on a healthier lifestyle plan? Finish the week with a powerful walk, walking toward your better life.

Exercise 6: Calf raise
4–6 reps, 2 sets

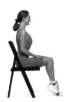

FEELING SCALE FOR EXERCISE
20 MAXIMUM EXERTION
19 EXTRA HARD
17 VERY HARD
16 HARDER
15 HARD
12 LIGHT
10 VERY LIGHT

Food for the day

Breakfast

Snack

Lunch
Monster salad, add vegetables and fruit, as well as the usual salad greens

Snack

Evening meal

Light snack

★ Goal for the week
Well, did you manage it?

★ Food goal
Have you tried steaming your vegetables?

Mood for the day
Mood at the start of the day
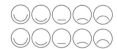
Mood at the end of the day

Fitness tips
Each time your brain tells you you can't make the last couple of reps, dip deep into your inner self. You probably can.

Motivation tips
Exercise gives you energy - you'll be able to pack so much more into your day.

WEEK SEVEN INTRODUCTION

This may feel initially like a hard week – you're nearly at the end of the second month, but not quite. If you feel in a sort of limbo, stop and think about how well you have done and how far you have come. Remind yourself of all the things you have discovered about yourself, of everything you have changed in your body, but also in your mind and your home and at work. Tell yourself how good you look and feel and enjoy the sensation each day of doing something positive for yourself.

Continue in the belief that each day you are a little step nearer your big goal. Setting small goals gives you the ability to succeed and do it well. Each one gives you the confidence to stride on and helps you not to worry about how much you weigh – feeling good physically and mentally is what living is all about. Eating good foods to fuel your body and exercising daily give your body what it wants. How's the food diary? Don't go slack on yourself; if you miss a day, try to work backward from the last meal you had and see if this helps. If not, just carry on from where you left off.

It is important for you to see what you have been doing over the last four weeks. At the end of next week it's assessment time. Your daily 15 minute walk should this week be firmly established in your routine. Each day set yourself a goal on your route: maybe the first day time yourself, the second, try to improve on this time, find a new route on day three, and so on. Make it a challenge and have some fun.

This week's exercise works the biceps, the muscle situated along the front of your arm from your shoulder joint to your elbow. So you're thinking 'I don't want bulging biceps': you won't get them. (If you do want them, you need to spend hours in the gym working heavy weights.) But every day you pick things up and carry them from one place to another. Why not make it easier to do that by strengthening these muscles.

This exercise, which complements the triceps extension you have been doing, will gradually improve the shape of your arms, giving them sleeker lines. For maximum benefit, watch your fat intake.

BICEP CURL

You can also do this exercise standing.

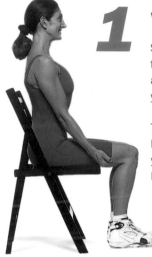

1

Warm up and stretch.

Sit with your knees and feet hip width apart and feet flat on the floor. Keep your back straight, ribcage lifted and tummy pulled in. Relax your shoulders and keep your head in line with your spine. Look forward.

Tuck your elbows in to your sides, next to your hip bones. Keeping your wrists straight, make a fist with your hands, but don't squeeze so tightly that your knuckles turn white.

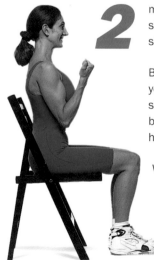

2

Breathe in, then as you breathe out, resist the arm movement and bring your hands up toward your shoulders. Keep your upper arms tucked into your sides as you do so.

Breathe in as you resist the movement down toward your thighs. Keep your upper arms in contact with your sides throughout. Focus your attention on the muscle being used, the more you resist the harder the muscle has to work. Take your time and do it well.

Work the stated number of repetitions and sets.

BICEP STRETCH

This is a difficult area to stretch and it may take you a few attempts to feel this stretch properly, but persevere – you will do it. This stretch can be done standing or sitting.

Breathe normally throughout.

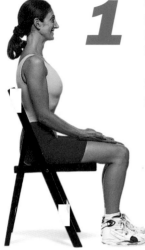

Sit with your knees and feet hip width apart and your feet flat on the floor. Keep your back straight, ribcage lifted and tummy pulled in. Relax your shoulders and keep your head in line with your spine. Look forward.

Place your hands palms up on your thighs; check that your shoulders are still relaxed.

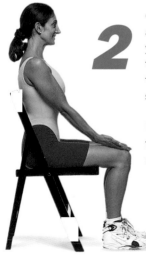

Gently press from your elbows into the fronts of your arms to straighten your arms but stop short of locking your elbow joints. Feel the gentle stretch running through the front of your arm, from your shoulder joint to your elbow; try to visualize the muscle you are stretching.

Hold the stretch for 8–10 seconds when you warm up, for 20–30 seconds as part of your cool down, then relax.

Fitness for the day
Walk 15 mins

You have reached 3 sets of leg extensions, congratulations. Continue to work on improving your posture while you are exercising and walking. Make each repetition and each set count, remember that the last few repetitions of any set are important in order to overload the muscle, which you must do to develop strength and definition, and to stimulate your body to burn the fuel you give it and the fat you are storing.

Exercise 1: Wall press
16–18 reps, 3 sets
Exercise 2: Leg extension
reps 14–16 reps, 3 sets
Exercise 3: Lower abdomen
raise 12–14 reps, 2 sets
Exercise 4: Tricep extension
10–12 reps, 2 sets
Exercise 5: Shoulder shrug
8–10 reps, 2 sets

FEELING SCALE FOR EXERCISE

20 MAXIMUM EXERTION

19 EXTRA HARD

17 VERY HARD

16 HARDER

15 HARD

12 LIGHT

10 VERY LIGHT

Food for the day

Breakfast

Snack

Lunch
Spiced potato bake – add chopped spinach, pine kernels and cumin or nutmeg

Snack

Evening meal

Light snack

★ Goal for the week
Have you checked out the leisure centre? How about making that a goal?

★ Fitness goal
To make every repetition count.

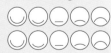

Mood for the day
Mood at the start of the day ◡ ◡ ◡ ◡ ◡
Mood at the end of the day ◡ ◡ ◡ ◡ ◡

Food tips
Fresh and unrefined foods really are the best for you.

Motivation tips
Changing how you think will change how you feel. Honestly.

Fitness for the day
Walk 15 mins

You will now be finding your walks easier, less demanding on your heart and lungs, because you have stimulated your body into feeling good, and each day that you go out walking, you improve your body's ability to keep going comfortably. Walk with attitude, enjoy yourself – and keep checking your posture.

★ Food goal

Have you kicked the packet of crisps/salted peanuts/biscuits/cake/ habit that is firmly entrenched?

FEELING SCALE FOR EXERCISE

20 MAXIMUM EXERTION

19 EXTRA HARD

17 VERY HARD

16 HARDER

15 HARD

12 LIGHT

10 VERY LIGHT

Food for the day

Breakfast

Snack

Lunch

Sheep's yogurt heaped with fresh fruit salad

Snack

Evening meal

Light snack

★ Goal for the week

Are you going to make it?

Mood for the day

Mood at the start of the day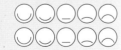

Mood at the end of the day

Fitness tips

Remind yourself how good you felt during your walk.

Motivation tips

You hold the controls – think positive.

WEEK SEVEN DAY THREE

Fitness for the day

Aim for the maximum number of repetitions you can do comfortably. Feel the muscles working, check your posture and enjoy the movement of your muscles as you work them. Remember to resist both upward and downward movements so that these exercises enhance your shape.

Exercise 1: Wall press
16–18 reps, 3 sets
Exercise 2: Leg extension
14–16 reps, 3 sets
Exercise 3: Lower abdomen raise
12–14 reps, 2 sets
Exercise 4: Tricep extension
10–12 reps, 2 sets
Exercise 5: Shoulder shrug
8–10 reps, 2 sets

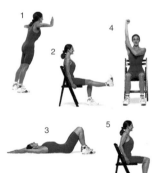

FEELING SCALE FOR EXERCISE

20 MAXIMUM EXERTION

19 EXTRA HARD

17 VERY HARD

16 HARDER

15 HARD

12 LIGHT

10 VERY LIGHT

Food for the day

Breakfast

Summer porridge - oats with freshly juiced strawberry, raspberry or blackcurrant juice

Snack

Lunch

Snack

Evening meal

Light snack

★ Goal for the week

Still feeling good?

★ Fitness goal

To walk the children to school.

Mood for the day

Mood at the start of the day

Mood at the end of the day

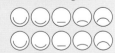

Food tips

Buy some fresh herbs and keep them on the window sill. They will add flavour to everything you eat.

Motivation tips

Do the best you can; it's all you can do.

Fitness for the day
Walk 15 mins

The improvements in your fitness level are subtle and you may not have noticed how much more able, more mobile and agile you are. Are you less tired? Better able to cope? How much energy do you have? Can you walk upstairs comfortably? It is these little changes that make all the difference.

★ Food goal

Have you cooked a new recipe this week? How about that for today's goal?

FEELING SCALE FOR EXERCISE

20
MAXIMUM EXERTION

19
EXTRA HARD

17
VERY HARD

16
HARDER

15
HARD

12
LIGHT

10
VERY LIGHT

Food for the day

Breakfast

Snack

Lunch

Snack
Cereal bar, but read the label and watch the fat and sugar content

Evening meal

Light snack

★ Goal for the week

Take no notice of others, unless they are positively encouraging.

Mood for the day

Mood at the start of the day

Mood at the end of the day

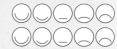

Fitness tips
Regular exercise three or four times a week will maintain your current level of fitness.

Motivation tips
Keep at it – this will soon feel like your normal lifestyle.

Fitness for the day
Walk 15 mins

A new exercise today to work your biceps (the muscles at the front of your arms). Take your time and make every movement precise, feel the resistance both upward and downward. Keep your elbows close in to your body, relax your shoulders and make your arm muscles do the work. Reread the coaching points for the calf raises to be sure your feet are in the right place.

Exercise 6:
Calf raise 6–8 reps, 2 sets
Exercise 7:
Bicep curl 4–6 reps, 1 sets

FEELING SCALE FOR EXERCISE

20 MAXIMUM EXERTION

19 EXTRA HARD

17 VERY HARD

16 HARDER

15 HARD

12 LIGHT

10 VERY LIGHT

Food for the day

Breakfast

Snack

Lunch

Snack

Evening meal
Grilled chicken basted with mint (fresh from your windowsill or garden) and yogurt

Light snack

★ Goal for the week
How's it going?

★ Fitness goal
To try one new leisure activity.

Mood for the day
Mood at the start of the day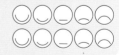
Mood at the end of the day

Food tips
Wash fruit and vegetables before eating or cooking. Buy organic whenever you can.

Motivation tips
Keep occupied, keep moving, keep healthy.

Fitness for the day
Walk 15 mins

This is so good, well done.
Remember to use your
arms, pumping from your
shoulders, through your
elbows into your hands.
Keep your hips square to
the front and walk tall.
If you become bored with
your route, change it.
Change direction, go a
different way, but whatever
you do, do it well, keeping
up the pace.

★ Food goal

Turn the whole family on to
fresh juice – you and they will
never look back.

FEELING SCALE FOR EXERCISE

20
MAXIMUM EXERTION

19
EXTRA HARD

17
VERY HARD

16
HARDER

15
HARD

12
LIGHT

10
VERY LIGHT

Food for the day

Breakfast

Snack

Lunch

Snack
Rice cakes with sugar-free jam

Evening meal

Light snack

★ Goal for the week
Are you going to make it?

Mood for the day

Mood at the
start of the day

Mood at the end
of the day

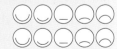

Fitness tips
When you feel yourself tensing,
relax, let your arms swing freely from
your shoulders.

Motivation tips
You are on to a winner. Keep your
willpower.

Fitness for the day
Walk 15 mins

You have done brilliantly, continue in this frame of mind, don't worry about setbacks, get straight back into it.

This is the second day of your second group of exercises, and you are looking good. Are you fitting it all in? Do as much as you can and take it slowly so that, like your walking, your workouts become part of your life. You're into week 8 tomorrow and the end of the second month. You have proven to yourself that, if you make an effort, you can exercise, walk, improve your eating habits and generally lift your moods. Go for it.

Exercise 6: Calf raise
6–8 reps, 2 sets
Exercise 7: Bicep curl
4–6 reps, 2 sets

6   7

★ Fitness goal
Climbed any stairs yet this week?

FEELING SCALE FOR EXERCISE

20
MAXIMUM EXERTION

19
EXTRA HARD

17
VERY HARD

16
HARDER

15
HARD

12
LIGHT

10
VERY LIGHT

Food for the day

Breakfast

Snack

Lunch

Snack

Evening meal
Fish (cod or another chunky white fish) and vegetable kebabs, served with rice

Light snack

★ Goal for the week
So, are you feeling pleased with yourself?

Mood for the day
Mood at the start of the day
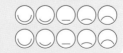
Mood at the end of the day

Food tips
Put down your knife and fork between mouthfuls. Make conversation, sip chilled water. Meals are social occasions.

Motivation tips
If you don't feel good about your body, you can't feel good about yourself. Keep at it.

WEEK EIGHT INTRODUCTION

Week 8 – wow! You have almost completed your second month, the second step on your road to fitness. You must be feeling proud of yourself. You have shown immense dedication and self-belief, hopefully without too many setbacks along the way. You have come a long way since week 1. It is so important to remember why you are doing this and to consider how the benefits of good foods and exercise, along with daily walks, have affected you.

At the end of this week it's assessment time again (turn to pp. 113–14), time to put on those articles of clothing that you are using as your guide to how you are changing shape gradually, or get out the tape measure and find out. Your clothes should be feeling more comfortable and fitting you looser. You should be feeling pretty good.

Add up all those mood faces and get a clearer picture of how you have been feeling for the last month. Were you affected by your moods? Did they improve? How did your workouts and walking affect you? Have a look and see for yourself.

Your food diary should be looking pretty full and very interesting. Is there a pattern here? Were your moods affected by what you ate and drank? Look and see for yourself. How much fat have you been accumulating over the weeks? Is there room for improvement here? Do you need to set yourself some new goals? Or do you need to continue with the same ones? Is the eating pattern changing? Treat each day as a new challenge – you know you can set goals and achieve them. Stay with it – there is only the last step to go, so go for it.

Continue to look at and read the coaching points for all the exercises, not simply the new ones each week. You should be getting stronger by the day and feeling that you have more control of your movements and are better able to do the things you want to do. Are there certain stretches or exercises you feel have improved quite noticeably? This will differ for everyone. If you are still finding some or all hard, persevere and you will break through.

This week's exercise is for your hamstrings, the muscles at the back of your upper thighs which easily weaken if not used – if you drive everywhere or sit at a desk all day and never take the stairs. Working your hamstrings balances the work you have been doing on your quadriceps (the muscles at the front of your thighs, see pp. 42–3). Remember that you must work toward equal strength in the muscles in both the front and back of each part of your body – they all work together. If you do not pay attention to this, or any other, major muscle group, you are setting yourself up for problems in later life.

HAMSTRING CURL

This exercise can be performed lying down with your hips firmly pressed into the floor, or standing as here. If you stand, use a chair for support.

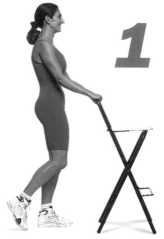

1 Warm up and stretch.

Stand facing the chair with your legs hip width apart and feet facing forward.

Place your hands on the back of the chair, shoulder width apart.

Keep your back straight, ribcage lifted and tummy pulled in. Relax your shoulders and keep your head in line with your spine. Look forward.

2 Soften your knees slightly (so that they are not locked). Tilt your pelvis forward slightly so that it is in line with your body.

Take a deep breath in and out. Breathe in again and this time, as you breathe out, curl the toes of your right foot toward your shin. Check your posture, then leading with the heel of your right foot, resist and curl your foot toward your buttocks. Keep your buttocks tight so that your hips are stable.

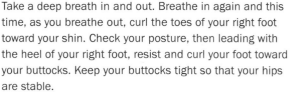

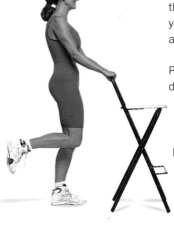

Pause as you squeeze into the back of your thigh and deep into the muscle. You may need to lean forward slightly to keep the back straight.

Breathe in as you draw your foot back toward the floor, pressing through your heel and leading through the toes. As your toes touch the floor, slowly and under resistance, repeat.

Work one set of the stated number of repetitions, then repeat using your other leg. Work the stated number of reps and sets with both legs.

HAMSTRING STRETCH

This is a good stretch at any time, not simply before and after exercise. Don't worry about how far you can get your leg over your head – this is not a competitive activity; you are stretching and relaxing your body for you. Remember that you are unique.

Breathe normally throughout.

Lie on your back, bend both your knees and place your feet hip width apart and flat on the floor.

Your neck should be completely relaxed and in line with your spine – you may like a cushion for added comfort.

Raise your right knee toward your chest and place your hands behind your thigh.

To ensure that your back stays flat to the floor, slowly slide your left foot forward a fraction or two. As you do so, feel your lower back coming into contact with the floor. Hold this position.

Very gently, as you extend your right leg, slide your hands toward the back of your knee. When you feel mild – but comfortable – tension in the back of your thigh, hold it.

If you find this difficult, your hamstrings really are tight or short. If your leg is shaking or trembling, ease back on the stretch a little. You may need to place a towel around your ankle and use this as an extension to your arms, so that you can feel the stretch in the back of your thigh, not in your neck!

Hold the stretch for 8–10 seconds when you warm up, for 20–30 seconds as part of your cool down, then relax.

Repeat using your other leg.

Fitness for the day
Walk 15 mins

You are now up to three sets of lower abs raises – well done. It may seem a little difficult at first, but you and your body will soon get used to it. Work hard to get good results.

Exercise 1: Wall press 18–20 reps, 3 sets
Exercise 2: Leg extension 16–18 reps, 3 sets
Exercise 3: Lower abdomen raise 14–16 reps, 3 sets
Exercise 4: Tricep extension 12–14 reps, 2 sets
Exercise 5: Shoulder shrug 10–12 reps, 2 sets

FEELING SCALE FOR EXERCISE

20 MAXIMUM EXERTION

19 EXTRA HARD

17 VERY HARD

16 HARDER

15 HARD

12 LIGHT

10 VERY LIGHT

Food for the day

Breakfast

Snack

Lunch

Snack
Hot tuna and mustard on toast

Evening meal

Light snack

★ **Goal for the week**
Think carefully about what you want to achieve.

★ **Food goal**
To leave the butter in the packet.

Mood for the day

Mood at the start of the day

Mood at the end of the day

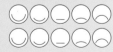

Fitness tips
Sit at your desk with your tummy in and back straight. Can't you breathe more easily?

Motivation tips
Don't feel guilty about an off day. Just do more tomorrow.

Fitness for the day
Walk 15-16 mins

Well done, you're over the halfway mark on the walking programme. Taking this time out is important for your health, your weight control, the way you feel and the way you look. Respect this time. Go out and walk hard, give your body a workout, pump those arms and blast away those cobwebs.

★ Fitness goal
Think carefully about what you want to achieve.

FEELING SCALE FOR EXERCISE

20
MAXIMUM
EXERTION

19
EXTRA
HARD

17
VERY
HARD

16
HARDER

15
HARD

12
LIGHT

10
VERY
LIGHT

Food for the day

Breakfast

Snack

Lunch

Jacket potato loaded with vegetable curry

Snack

Evening meal

Light snack

★ Goal for the week
How's it going?

Mood for the day

Mood at the start of the day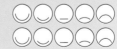

Mood at the end of the day

Food tips
Soak a huge pot of mixed beans overnight, then while you eat breakfast, boil them up. They will keep for days in the fridge, for salads, casseroles and snacks.

Motivation tips
Refusal and rejection are not the same things.

Fitness for the day
Walk 16 mins

Push for the maximum number of repetitions on all exercises and all sets. Take time to do them well. There is no point in rushing the workout and forfeiting your technique. You have the whole of your life to sculpture your body and change the world. Play safe, stay injury free, learn gradually and painlessly.

Exercise 1: Wall press
18–20 reps, 3 sets
Exercise 2: Leg extension
16–18 reps, 3 sets
Exercise 3: Lower abdomen
raise 14–16 reps, 3 sets
Exercise 4: Tricep extension
12–14 reps, 2 sets
Exercise 5: Shoulder shrug
10–12 reps, 2 sets

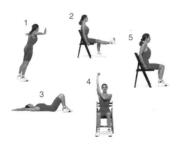

FEELING SCALE FOR EXERCISE

20
MAXIMUM EXERTION

19
EXTRA HARD

17
VERY HARD

16
HARDER

15
HARD

12
LIGHT

10
VERY LIGHT

Food for the day

Breakfast

Snack

Lunch

Snack

Evening meal

Mixed bean casserole – make it with onions, mushrooms, vegetable stock and any vegetables you like

Light snack

★ Goal for the week
Still feeling good?

★ Fitness goal
To try one new sporting activity.

Mood for the day

Mood at the start of the day
Mood at the end of the day

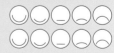

Fitness tips
Think posture – tummy in, head high, shoulders back, back straight.

Motivation tips
Life's a balancing act, but you can have everything if you want it enough.

Fitness for the day
Walk 16-17 mins

Rain or shine, you need to be walking, your body needs oxygen every day. If you really want to burn the food you are eating and the fat that firmly moulded itself to your beautiful body, your must get your basic level of daily activity up and stop putting in the excess fat and sugar. There is no other safe way – no other plan in the world will do for you what exercise and aerobic work can do.

★ Food goal

Have you cooked a new recipe this week? How about that for today's goal?

FEELING SCALE FOR EXERCISE

20
MAXIMUM EXERTION

19
EXTRA HARD

17
VERY HARD

16
HARDER

15
HARD

12
LIGHT

10
VERY LIGHT

Food for the day

Breakfast

Snack

Lunch

Snack
Low-fat fromage frais with fresh fruit

Evening meal

Light snack

★ Goal for the week

Remember how good you felt when you started the programme. Go forward from there.

Mood for the day

Mood at the start of the day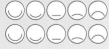

Mood at the end of the day

Fitness tips
Don't overheat yogurt or fromage frais – both will curdle.

Motivation tips
Believe in yourself – you can do this.

Fitness for the day
Walk 17 mins

Another exercise for the lower body this week, this one concentrating on the upper backs of your thighs. Read the coaching points carefully and study the photographs. Concentrate on working the muscle through its whole range of movement and resist in both directions, upward and downward. Visualize the shape you want your thighs to be.

Exercise 6: Calf raise
8–10 reps, 2 sets
Exercise 7: Bicep curl
6–8 reps, 2 sets
Exercise 8: Hamstring curl
4–6 reps, 1 set

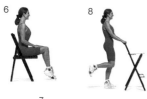

FEELING SCALE FOR EXERCISE

20 MAXIMUM EXERTION

19 EXTRA HARD

17 VERY HARD

16 HARDER

15 HARD

12 LIGHT

10 VERY LIGHT

Food for the day

Breakfast

Snack

Lunch

Egg white omelette with mixed vegetables - add dried fruits, nuts and seeds if you like too

Snack

Evening meal

Light snack

★ Goal for the week
Still on target?

★ Food goal
To drink more water to flush out toxins.

Mood for the day

Mood at the start of the day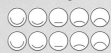

Mood at the end of the day

Fitness tips
Visualize the muscles you want and feel them becoming firmer.

Motivation tips
Be true to yourself.

Fitness for the day
Walk 17-18 mins

Get those happy hormones pumping. Walk tall, check your posture and make your arms do some serious work. More oxygen to your body and your brain will release endorphins into your system, giving you a sense of euphoria, a natural high, that can do wonders for your sex life.

★ Fitness goal

If you can't decide, see if you can run to the bus stop or station.

FEELING SCALE FOR EXERCISE

20 MAXIMUM EXERTION

19 EXTRA HARD

17 VERY HARD

16 HARDER

15 HARD

12 LIGHT

10 VERY LIGHT

Food for the day

Breakfast

Toast with vegemite and grilled tomatoes

Snack

Lunch

Snack

Evening meal

Light snack

★ Goal for the week

Are you going to make it?

Mood for the day

Mood at the start of the day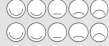

Mood at the end of the day

Food tips

Trim off all visible fat.

Motivation tips

Self discipline is the foundation of self improvement.

Fitness for the day
Walk 18-20 mins

You should be feeling very pleased with how well you have done, how good you are looking, and how good you feel. Today spend some time looking over the last month. Do your assessment for the month, filling in the charts on pp. 113–14. Put your measuring clothes on and feel the difference. How much looser are they? How much firmer are you? On to week 9.

Exercise 6:
Calf raise 8–10 reps, 2 sets
Exercise 7:
Bicep curl 6–8 reps, 2 sets
Exercise 8:
Hamstring curl 4–6 reps, 2 sets

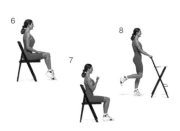

FEELING SCALE FOR EXERCISE

20
MAXIMUM EXERTION

19
EXTRA HARD

17
VERY HARD

16
HARDER

15
HARD

12
LIGHT

10
VERY LIGHT

Food for the day

Breakfast

Snack

Lunch

Snack

Evening meal

Grilled salmon with lemon juice and fresh dill, new potatoes and a large salad

Light snack

★ Goal for the week
Did you make it?

★ Food goal
Aim to find an alternative family treat to burgers and fries.

Mood for the day
Mood at the start of the day
Mood at the end of the day

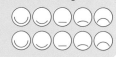

Fitness tips
Don't worry about the next set; concentrate on this one.

Motivation tips
Don't act on the wishes and expectations of others – it is you who counts.

Have you tried on the item you are using to measure your weight loss? If you have you will probably be pleasantly surprised since two months of improved diet and regular exercise have almost certainly made a difference. It is now time to fill in the grids and note here the improvement over the past month.

Fitness and food assessment

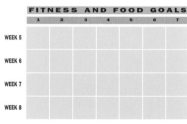

At the end of each week add up how many times you reached your goal and note it on the grid. Did you achieve more goals in week eight than week five? How about looking back at week one and noting the improvement over these weeks? Is it getting easier? Do you feel less tired, better able to cope? Is your improved diet making a difference to how you feel? Have any new foods become part of your repertoire?

6–7 goals per week
This is excellent, but are you perhaps making them a bit easy? Try an extra set or a couple more repetitions. Try to wean yourself off something that is really proving hard.

4–5 goals per week
Very good. Try not to fall below this level; push yourself but keep it realistic – you are well on the way. Are food or fitness goals contributing to this good score; if one or the other takes precedence, aim for equal success with both.

3 goals per week
Good. Three is better than two and next month you may well be up to four or five – keep at it.

1–2 goals per week
Keep trying. Don't be beaten. Lighten up a little and make your goals a bit easier next week – you will get there. Remember that people respond to changes in different ways. Check your vulnerable times in the diary and work on them. This could be responsible for big improvements next month.

ASSESSMENT

Feeling scale assessment

Add up the entries on your feeling scales and note them on the grid. Are you reaching 15–16–17 at least five times a week when your exercise? Most people work for too long at too low an intensity – be aware of this as you exercise. Try not to slip below 15.

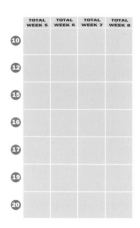

	TOTAL WEEK 5	TOTAL WEEK 6	TOTAL WEEK 7	TOTAL WEEK 8
10				
12				
15				
16				
17				
19				
20				

Mood scale assessment

Fill in the mood grids for the beginning and end of each day. Are your moods improving overall? How many days do you wake up feeling good and stay that way all day? In time these days will be in the majority, even if that now seems unrealistic. Keep at it – you will get there.

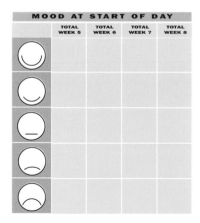

MOOD AT START OF DAY	TOTAL WEEK 5	TOTAL WEEK 6	TOTAL WEEK 7	TOTAL WEEK 8
🙂				
🙂				
😐				
🙁				
☹️				

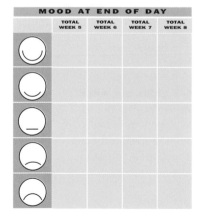

MOOD AT END OF DAY	TOTAL WEEK 5	TOTAL WEEK 6	TOTAL WEEK 7	TOTAL WEEK 8
🙂				
🙂				
😐				
🙁				
☹️				

WEEK NINE INTRODUCTION

Here you go into week 9 and the third month. Congratulations – you are doing magnificently well. Didn't the end-of-month assessment make good reading? Focus your attention on the week ahead, when we will be concentrating on making your 20-minute walk a powerful one: aim for 16–17 on the feeling scale every day. Pump your arms and really stride out to increase your heart rate, to pump more oxygen to your working muscles. Visualize your body's metabolic rate increasing as you walk every day and make more effort every day. Stay with it – you are doing fabulously!

Your walk should by now be cemented in your daily routine, and you have no doubts whatever that it makes you feel good. Did you score well in the end-of-month assessment? Is it time to change some goals and up the tempo a bit? Or are you happy to make sure that you really do reach your one goal? Achieving a goal makes you feel so good, and you know now that – as long as you keep your goals small and realistic – you will continue to achieve them.

In the course of this week, you will as usual work more sets and reps than last week, so that exercise 4 (the triceps extension) is now up to three sets, congratulations. Remember to resist the upward and downward movements on all the exercises. This week's new exercise is the shoulder press. The shoulder area is another one of those that rarely get worked: when did you last raise or push your arms over your head? Yet it is important to have some tone here. You need strength in these muscles, just as you do in any others – remember that weak muscles become weaker and stronger muscles become stressed. As you ask your arms and upper body to lift and carry heavy objects, you put stress not only on your upper body, but also on your lower back and, perhaps, further down your body.

This exercise may appear difficult at first, but persevere and, like any other muscle, this will become stronger with time and effort. The weaker the muscle, the more you need to focus on ensuring correct technique and challenging yourself to complete all the repetitions and all the sets. Generally, your upper body responds quite quickly to any increase in workload. So by doing this exercise you will start to see and feel a difference in your appearance, which is psychologically important. Also, you tend to store less fat here which means that it is easier to see the results of all your efforts.

You have done excellently – keep at it.

SHOULDER PRESS

This exercise can be worked standing, but I have chosen to sit as this makes you more stable and therefore better able to focus on what you are doing.

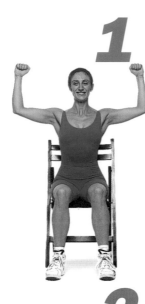

1

Warm up and stretch.

Sit with your back straight, ribcage lifted and tummy pulled in. Relax your shoulders and keep your head in line with your spine. Look forward.

Start by working one arm (when you are happy with your technique, you can work both at the same time, as shown). Be sure to keep your back upright, don't allow it to arch.

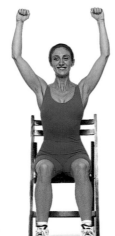

2

Keeping both your shoulders facing the front, breathe in and out deeply. Make a fist with your working arm and hold your arm out at the side of your body as shown in the picture.

Breathe in, then as you breathe out, press your fist upward. Imagine you are moving it through treacle or mud and resist the air. Stop short of locking your elbow, pause, then start to lower your arm, again resisting the air as if you were moving through something thick and sticky.

Pause and repeat. Work a set with one arm, then repeat using your other arm. Work the stated number of repetitions and sets with both arms.

SHOULDER STRETCH

You can stand or sit to work this stretch, but whichever you choose keep your back straight.

Breathe normally throughout.

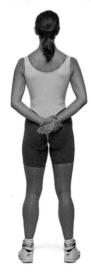

1 With your back straight, put both hands behind your back.

With your left hand take hold of your right wrist.

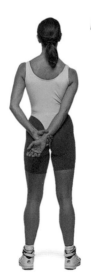

2 Very slowly and gently pull on your right wrist. Feel the stretch up into the top of your shoulder and neck – this is a fabulous stretch for this area.

Hold for the stated number of seconds, making sure your posture is good, then gently let go of your wrist.

Stretch for 8–10 seconds when you warm up, for 20–30 seconds as part of your cool down, then relax. Repeat right ear to right shoulder.

Fitness for the day
Walk 20 mins

You are now so familiar with these exercises that you can concentrate on putting more effort into them. But never, at any stage, let your posture slip. Keep your body upright, and you will truly benefit in your everyday life. You should be feeling stronger and more in control of your movements, and enjoying the benefits that brings. Stay in touch with your muscles as you do the exercises, it really helps to visualize the muscle working: make an effort and do the repetitions slowly.

Exercise 1: Wall press
20–22 reps, 3 sets
Exercise 2: Leg extension
18–20 reps, 3 sets
Exercise 3: Lower abdomen
raise 16–18 reps, 3 sets
Exercise 4: Tricep extension
14–16 reps, 3 sets
Exercise 5: Shoulder shrug
12–14 reps, 2 sets

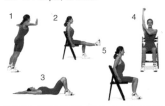

FEELING SCALE FOR EXERCISE

20 MAXIMUM EXERTION

19 EXTRA HARD

17 VERY HARD

16 HARDER

15 HARD

12 LIGHT

10 VERY LIGHT

Food for the day

Breakfast

Snack

Lunch
Cold grilled turkey with broccoli and apple salad

Snack

Evening meal

Light snack

★ Goal for the week
Have you booked a beginners' class at the local sports centre?

★ Fitness goal
To buy a kite and spend time in the fresh air flying it.

Mood for the day
Mood at the start of the day
Mood at the end of the day
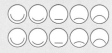

Food tips
Adapt favourite recipes to reduce fat content. Try halving the recommended amounts to start with.

Motivation tips
There is not one food or one habit that makes you overweight and out of condition – everything in moderation.

WEEK NINE DAY TWO

Fitness for the day
Walk 20 mins

The benefits of this 20-minute walk should now be shining through every day. Can you feel your body come to life as it enjoys taking in oxygen. Stride out and make it a good walk with lots of effort. Work your buttocks muscles, try to find a hill and challenge yourself to walk up it, squeezing and holding the tension in your muscles and focusing on working them hard.

★ Food goal

Count up all the hidden sugars you consume today – you will be surprised. Aim to half this by the end of the month.

FEELING SCALE FOR EXERCISE

20 MAXIMUM EXERTION

19 EXTRA HARD

17 VERY HARD

16 HARDER

15 HARD

12 LIGHT

10 VERY LIGHT

Food for the day

Breakfast

Snack

Lunch

Snack

Evening meal

Light snack

Rice cakes with chopped banana

★ Goal for the week

Take no notice of others, unless they are positively encouraging.

Mood for the day

Mood at the start of the day

Mood at the end of the day

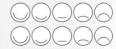

Fitness tips

Pump your arms, expand your lungs, feel the air doing you good.

Motivation tips

You may stimulate your metabolism more quickly or more slowly than someone else. Don't worry about it – just do it.

Fitness for the day
Walk 26 mins

Try standing slightly further away from the wall as you do your wall presses – not so far as to cause you to lose your posture and let your back start taking the strain, but enough to make your upper body have to work that bit harder. Try moving your arms slightly wider apart, too, but again be sensible. These slight changes will help you to challenge your body and to keep your mind on what you are doing.

Exercise 1: Wall press 20–22 reps, 3 sets
Exercise 2: Leg extension 18–20 reps, 3 sets
Exercise 3: Lower abdomen raise 16–18 reps, 3 sets
Exercise 4: Tricep extension 14–16 reps, 3 sets
Exercise 5: Shoulder shrug 12–14 reps, 2 sets

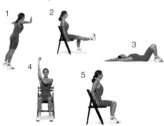

FEELING SCALE FOR EXERCISE

20 MAXIMUM EXERTION

19 EXTRA HARD

17 VERY HARD

16 HARDER

15 HARD

12 LIGHT

10 VERY LIGHT

Food for the day

Breakfast
Home-made muesli; note the ingredients you like in supermarket own brands, then mix those you prefer. Better your choice than someone else's

Snack

Lunch

Snack

Evening meal

Light snack

★ Goal for the week
Keep it up!

★ Fitness goal
To make every repetition count.

Mood for the day

Mood at the start of the day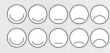

Mood at the end of the day

Food tips
Use fresh herbs instead of salt – delicious flavours and much healthier.

Motivation tips
You've come so far. Don't give up now.

Fitness for the day
Walk 20 mins

When walking today, think about all the changes that have occurred over the last nine weeks. Could you have walked like this at the beginning? Would your body have glowed with energy, during and after your walk and your exercises. Do you want to feel like this every day for the rest of your life? Stay fit for today and set yourself small obtainable goals each week, and the sense of euphoria from achieving them will enable you to look and feel as good as you do now.

★ Food goal

Have you cooked a new recipe this week? How about that for today's goal?

FEELING SCALE FOR EXERCISE

20 MAXIMUM EXERTION

19 EXTRA HARD

17 VERY HARD

16 HARDER

15 HARD

12 LIGHT

10 VERY LIGHT

Food for the day

Breakfast

Snack

Lunch

Snack
Fresh fruit, anything you choose

Evening meal

Light snack

★ Goal for the week

Don't lose heart - I'm sure you're doing fine!

Mood for the day

Mood at the start of the day

Mood at the end of the day

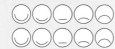

Fitness tips
Look around you as you walk; note the slight change in the season each day. Does it make you feel good?

Motivation tips
Walk for your future – get that heart pumping and keep your body glowing

Fitness for the day
Walk 20 mins

Today we add in another great exercise for the upper body. Concentrate on your posture and be sure to keep your abdominals in, your neck straight and shoulders square to the front. And – relax! How are you fitting the extra workout in? Are you managing the time? As with all the other efforts you have made over the weeks, I am sure that you will eventually fit it in, without having to think about it.

Exercise 6: Calf raise
10–12 reps, 2 sets 2
Exercise 7: Bicep curl
8–10 reps, 2 sets
Exercise 8: Hamstring curl
6–8 reps, 2 sets
Exercise 9: Shoulder press
4–6 reps, 1 set

6   7

8   9

FEELING SCALE FOR EXERCISE

20 MAXIMUM EXERTION

19 EXTRA HARD

17 VERY HARD

16 HARDER

15 HARD

12 LIGHT

10 VERY LIGHT

Food for the day

Breakfast

Freshly juiced oranges, add half a grapefruit to make slightly sharper, half an apple for more sweetness

Snack

Lunch

Snack

Evening meal

Light snack

★ Goal for the week
Still on target?

★ Fitness goal
To do an extra set when I'm feeling good.

Mood for the day

Mood at the start of the day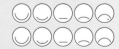

Mood at the end of the day

Food tips
Treat yourself to a new recipe book; aim to try one new recipe a week.

Motivation tips
If you don't enjoy yourself, nobody else will enjoy you either.

Fitness for the day
Walk 20 mins
You should be feeling stronger and fitter as you bound around your course. Aim for variety; perhaps after your warm-up walk, try fast walking between lamp posts or benches, vary the distance, walking fast between three lamp posts, slightly slower between the next two, and so on. And remember that the more brisk walking you do, the more you stimulate your body to burn.

★ Food goal
You don't have to join the Friday lunchtime session in the pub if you don't want to. How about giving it a miss this week?

FEELING SCALE FOR EXERCISE

20 MAXIMUM EXERTION

19 EXTRA HARD

17 VERY HARD

16 HARDER

15 HARD

12 LIGHT

10 VERY LIGHT

Food for the day

Breakfast

Snack

Lunch

Snack

Evening meal
Grilled chicken, marinated in yogurt and chives, with rice and steamed vegetables

Light snack

★ Goal for the week
Nearly there - don't give up.

Mood for the day
Mood at the start of the day
Mood at the end of the day

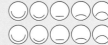

Fitness tips
Variety is the spice of life. Try something new – kite flying, yoga, swimming.

Motivation tips
If you don't enjoy yourself, nobody else will enjoy you either.

Fitness for the day
Walk 20 mins

Great work – you are now up to two sets of shoulder presses. Make the effort to do both sets equally well, don't rush the repetitions or sets, take your time and perform them with good technique. Weekly progression is the key here, you have to challenge your body to be able to improve upon it. If you don't challenge it, it will exert itself only enough for the task in hand. Work hard to make each repetition, each set and each walking session count.

Exercise 6: Calf raise
10–12 reps, 2 sets
Exercise 7: Bicep curl
8–10 reps, 2 sets
Exercise 8: Hamstring curl
6–8 reps, 2 sets
Exercise 9: Shoulder press
4–6 reps, 2 sets

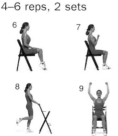

FEELING SCALE FOR EXERCISE
20 MAXIMUM EXERTION
19 EXTRA HARD
17 VERY HARD
16 HARDER
15 HARD
12 LIGHT
10 VERY LIGHT

Food for the day

Breakfast

Snack

Lunch

Snack

Grilled tomatoes on toast – snip fresh basil over the top

Evening meal

Light snack

★ Goal for the week
Did you make it?

★ Fitness goal
To walk an extra couple of minutes.

Mood for the day

Mood at the start of the day

Mood at the end of the day

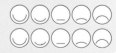

Food tips
If you want chocolate, buy the best quality you can find (that's the one with the highest percentage of cocoa solids). This is a once in a while treat, and you deserve the best.

Motivation tips
Congratulate yourself on your achievements – you are doing brilliantly.

WEEK TEN *INTRODUCTION*

O h boy! Am I excited for you! This is fantastic – week 10 already. How do you feel? Well enough to have reaped some of the rewards that true fitness can give you? I'm sure of that. This week might feel a bit hard, since it's a limbo week. If you find that, take a look back through the diary and remind yourself how well you are doing. Look in the mirror and see what is happening to you. Keep this in mind as you continue through the week.

This week we up the walk from 20 to 25 minutes – nearly at that magical 30. Concentrate on your walking and how well and how hard you are working. Focus your attention on your arm technique; remember to pump from your elbow up into your hand. Keep your elbows close to your body and your shoulders relaxed. Roll through your foot from heel to toe and keep checking your posture. Remember that this is not just important for your walking, it will also enhance how you stand and feel generally (see pp. 8–9).

This week you are focusing on your lower body, the legs that carry you everywhere. If you are carrying excess fat here, this exercise, daily walking and more aerobic work in general will help you to see improvements in the shape and feel of these muscles. This muscle group is one of the biggest, and works hard. This means that you have to work harder for good results. Remember that you have the rest of your life ahead of you. Stay with it and you will succeed. But it is going to be hard work.

How are your goals? How did they go last week? If you are having trouble reaching your weekly goals, perhaps you are making them too difficult, taking on too much at the moment. Think about it, reread pp. 10–13 and set yourself something that you can achieve this week. We all have bad days and weeks, so forget the past and think of the future.

CHAIR SQUAT

These squats can be performed without the chair, and eventually you will be able to do this, but I have incorporated it at this stage to be certain that you master the correct technique. Choose a chair that enables you to sit with your feet flat on the floor.

As you become stronger, try only to touch the chair with your buttocks between repetitions and do not sit. After six or seven weeks, try putting the chair at the side of you for support and balance. Never take a squat lower than seat height and always check your posture.

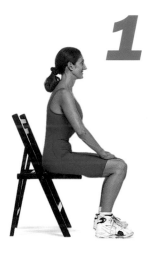

Warm up and stretch.

Sit with your knees and feet hip width apart (if your feet are together, your balance will be upset) and your feet flat on the floor

Keep your back straight, ribcage lifted and lower and upper abdominals pulled in. Relax your shoulders and keep your head in line with your spine. Look forward.

Rest your hands on the front of your thighs, and focus your attention on the muscles you are about to use. Really concentrate on both phases of the exercise.

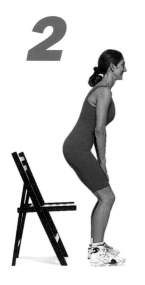

Breathe in, then as you breathe out, slowly stand up using your legs, not your back. Press your heels firmly into the floor as you press up through them into your calves and the back and front of your upper legs and finally – as you approach a standing position – your buttock muscles. Squeeze deeply.

Tilt your hips forward slightly. Pause at this point, squeezing into your buttock muscles. Breathe in as you lower your buttocks toward the seat. Resist the downward movement, as if you were moving through treacle or mud.

When you reach the start position, check your posture, then repeat. Work the stated number of repetitions and sets.

BUTTOCKS STRETCH

Breathe normally throughout.

1 Lie flat on your back, with your knees bent and hip width apart, and your feet flat on the floor.

Make sure that your back is pressed firmly into the floor and that your head is in line with your spine.

2 Bring your right knee toward your chest, placing your right foot on your left knee. If you find it difficult to get comfortable in this position, and/or your back is arching, slowly slide your left foot forward a little. As you do so, feel your back lengthen, and your lower back come into contact with the floor. There should not be any pressure around your knee.

Hold this position for 8–10 seconds when you warm up, for 20–30 seconds as part of your cool down, then relax.

Fitness for the day
Walk 20 mins

All five exercises are now on three sets, that's great! Your body is showing positive signs of improvements, which should make you feel stronger and more confident. Stay focused on each exercise, each repetition and each set. If you are finding some of these exercises easy, increase the repetitions, then the number of sets. Also try doing each repetition a little slower and really focus on resisting the movement upward and downward.

Exercise 1: Wall press 22–24 reps, 3 sets
Exercise 2: Leg extension 20–22 reps, 3 sets
Exercise 3: Lower abdomen raise 18–20 reps, 3 sets
Exercise 4: Tricep extension 18–20 reps, 3 sets
Exercise 5: Shoulder shrug 14–16 reps, 3 sets

FEELING SCALE FOR EXERCISE

20 MAXIMUM EXERTION

19 EXTRA HARD

17 VERY HARD

16 HARDER

15 HARD

12 LIGHT

10 VERY LIGHT

Food for the day

Breakfast

Snack

Lunch

Snack
Cottage cheese and pineapple granary roll

Evening meal

Light snack

★ Goal for the week
How about something really different this week?

★ Food goal
To treat my tastebuds.

Mood for the day

Mood at the start of the day

Mood at the end of the day

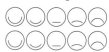

Fitness tips
Think tall, walk tall and enjoy today.

Motivation tips
Old habits are hard to change, new ones easy to adopt.

Fitness for the day
Walk 20-21 mins

Over the 20-minute mark – now we are really talking business. Gradually increase the pace, and keep your chest up. Let it expand so that your lungs fill up with oxygen. Work toward the 15–16–17 range of the feeling scale, encouraging your heart to pump harder, get those arms up and powering from your shoulders. Challenge yourself by stimulating your mind and your body.

★ Fitness goal

To keep trainers or walking shoes in the office and jog and walk in the park at lunchtime.

FEELING SCALE FOR EXERCISE

20
MAXIMUM EXERTION

☐

19
EXTRA HARD

☐

17
VERY HARD

☐

16
HARDER

☐

15
HARD

☐

12
LIGHT

☐

10
VERY LIGHT

Food for the day

Breakfast

Warm home-made lemon muffins

Snack

Lunch

Snack

Evening meal

Light snack

★ Goal for the week

Are you going to make it?

Mood for the day

Mood at the start of the day

Mood at the end of the day

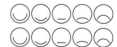

Food tips
Always check food labels for fat and sugar contents. You need no more than 30g (1oz) of fat a day, and some experts suggest less than this.

Motivation tips
You hold the controls as to how you think and act. Take charge.

Fitness for the day
Walk 21 mins

Try to do the maximum number of reps today as you complete all three sets of all five exercises, to bring you a little closer to your goals. Take your time and make every effort count. There is no point in wasting all this time.

Exercise 1: Wall press 22–24 reps, 3 sets
Exercise 2: Leg extension 20–22 reps, 3 sets
Exercise 3: Lower abdomen raise 18–20 reps, 3 sets
Exercise 4: Tricep extension 16–18 reps, 3 sets
Exercise 5: Shoulder shrug 14–16 reps, 3 sets

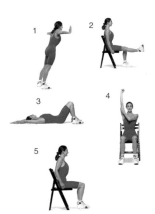

FEELING SCALE FOR EXERCISE

20 MAXIMUM EXERTION

19 EXTRA HARD

17 VERY HARD

16 HARDER

15 HARD

12 LIGHT

10 VERY LIGHT

Food for the day

Breakfast

Snack

Lunch
Ratatouille – but go easy on the oil and load up with the vegetables

Snack

Evening meal

Light snack

★ Goal for the week
Still on target?

★ Food goal
To eat at least three portions of fruit or vegetables a day.

Mood for the day

Mood at the start of the day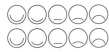

Mood at the end of the day

Fitness tips
Spend one more minute, do one more repetition and praise yourself afterward.

Motivation tips
Time spent on yourself is always worth while.

Fitness for the day
Walk 21-22 mins

There is that extra minute again! It's amazing how quickly you approach the next full 5 minutes. Keep up the good work and the high spirits you should be feeling. Walk with confidence, in the knowledge that you are working toward a better lifestyle, able to breathe comfortably and move properly. You are only as young as you feel – how old do you feel today?

★ Fitness goal

Do you walk an extra stop before catching the bus or train? Would that be a good goal?

FEELING SCALE FOR EXERCISE

20
MAXIMUM EXERTION

19
EXTRA HARD

17
VERY HARD

16
HARDER

15
HARD

12
LIGHT

10
VERY LIGHT

Food for the day

Breakfast

Snack

Lunch

Snack

Evening meal
Pasta in yogurt and tomato sauce with tuna and olives

Light snack

★ Goal for the week
Still feeling good?

Mood for the day

Mood at the start of the day

Mood at the end of the day

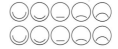

Food tips
Try one new food a week; you will be surprised how many you like.

Motivation tips
Exercising is more fun than television.

Fitness for the day
Walk 22 mins

Today we add in chair squats – fabulous exercise for the legs and buttocks. You really need to focus on the muscles of your buttocks here, and try to keep some tension in them as you sit down, and as you stand up. Expect some slight discomfort (not pain) as you train your brain and your body into accepting a new you. It can take some time, but take it easy and stick with it. You're nearly there. Well done.

Exercise 6: Calf raise
12–14 reps, 2 sets
Exercise 7: Bicep curl
10–12 reps, 2 sets
Exercise 8: Hamstring curl
8–10 reps, 2 sets
Exercise 9: Shoulder press
6–8 reps, 2 sets
Exercise 10: Chair squat
4–6 reps, 1 set

FEELING SCALE FOR EXERCISE

20 MAXIMUM EXERTION

19 EXTRA HARD

17 VERY HARD

16 HARDER

15 HARD

12 LIGHT

10 VERY LIGHT

Food for the day

Breakfast

Snack

Lunch
Mixed salad, as much as you can eat, with dressing made from orange juice and fresh coriander

Snack

Evening meal

Light snack

★ Goal for the week
Are you nearly there?

★ Food goal
To treat my tastebuds.

Mood for the day

Mood at the start of the day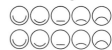

Mood at the end of the day

Fitness tips
Don't worry about the next set. Concentrate on the set in hand and do them well.

Motivation tips
A rest day is not the beginning of the end.

Fitness for the day
Walk 22-23 mins

How are you feeling? You should be really pleased with yourself for achieving this daily walk. Keep posture checking as you go, try to pay attention to how you are walking. When you pass another walker or jogger, say 'Hi, Hello, Morning, Afternoon, Evening'. Smile as you pass and feel the buzz from being outside and doing this for yourself.

★ Food goal
How about going without that packet of crisps on the way home?

FEELING SCALE FOR EXERCISE

20 MAXIMUM EXERTION

19 EXTRA HARD

17 VERY HARD

16 HARDER

15 HARD

12 LIGHT

10 VERY LIGHT

Food for the day

Breakfast

Wholemeal pancakes with lemon and maple syrup

Snack

Lunch

Snack

Evening meal

Light snack

★ Goal for the week
Are you feeling proud of yourself – you certainly should be.

Mood for the day

Mood at the start of the day

Mood at the end of the day

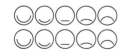

Food tips
Put the timer on when you are cooking porridge – why risk having it welded to the saucepan?

Motivation tips
Don't stop to question your success – get on and build on it!

Fitness for the day
Walk 23-25 mins

Two sets of chair squats today. Concentrate and keep checking the photographs and coaching points to make sure that your technique is correct and you are feeling the work in all the right places (your whole leg, including your buttocks). Aim for the full 25 minutes walk today. Look at this – two weeks to go. How do you feel?

Exercise 6: Calf raise
12–14 reps, 2 sets
Exercise 7: Biceps curl
10–12 reps, 2 sets
Exercise 8: Hamstring curl
8–10 reps, 2 sets
Exercise 9: Shoulder press
6–8 reps, 2 sets
Exercise 10: Chair squat
4–6 reps, 2 sets

FEELING SCALE FOR EXERCISE

20
MAXIMUM EXERTION

19
EXTRA HARD

17
VERY HARD

16
HARDER

15
HARD

12
LIGHT

10
VERY LIGHT

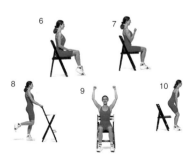

Food for the day
Breakfast

Snack

Lunch

Snack
Mixed dried fruits and unsalted nuts

Evening meal

Light snack

★ **Goal for the week**
Did you make it?

★ **Food goal**
Have you cooked a meatless meal?

Mood for the day
Mood at the start of the day
Mood at the end of the day

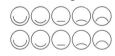

Fitness tips
Treat yourself to a new teeshirt or pair of joggers – you deserve it!

Motivation tips
Listen to your body – there is no one food that makes you fat, unhappy or depressed.

WEEK ELEVEN INTRODUCTION ➤

I bet this feels good! Aim to be as active as you can in your day-to-day activities and make a special effort this week to walk harder and farther. Try to set yourself a small goal when you are out on your walk. Since you broke the 20-minute mark, you should have noticed an increase in your stamina level.

This week is a challenge in itself, as you make the time to incorporate those last five minutes – from 25 to 30 – into your daily schedule. Try to make this a 16–17 week on the feeling scale so that your heart and lungs work a little harder. Get your body burning more fuel: remember that the more effort you put in, the better your results will be.

Make a special effort too with what you eat this week. Note which foods make you feel good, and which make you feel bad and/or hungry for more. You do want your last assessment to be good so that you can carry on and feel proud of what you have done, don't you?

Work hard at all the exercises, making each repetition as good as the last. Take your time and do them well. This week's new exercise is for those abdominals that run from under your breastbone, down to your pelvis. The underlying muscles of your abdomen will increase in tone and feel firmer to the touch through this exercise. Unfortunately, layers of swollen fat cells will wobble over the top and feel more loose so cut down on your intake of fats and sugars (be specially conscious of hidden ones), and up your basic daily activity level, anything to increase your metabolic rate so that you burn fat even when you are not exercising.

ABDOMINAL CURLS

This exercise is not easy, as you tend to want to pull on your neck in order to work the muscle deeper. Don't – all you will succeed in doing is putting stress on your neck and shoulders. The movement involved in lifting your chest off the floor is small: you must focus on using the muscles of your abdomen. Pay attention to the coaching points and concentrate on the muscles you are using.

 Warm up and stretch.

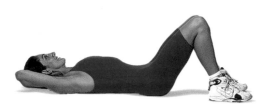

Lie on your back, bend both knees and place your feet hip width apart and flat on the floor. Place both hands over your head and down toward your shoulder blades (not too far, just at the nape of your neck) one on top of the other.

Relax your head into your hands and let them support you like a pillow. Imagine that you have a large orange under your chin – if you look down, you will squeeze the juice out and if you look up, it will roll away. Hold it so that your head is relaxed and you are not pulling on your neck.

Tilt your pelvis so that your lower back is firmly pressed into the floor.

Breathe in and out, then in again. This time, as you breathe out, press your lower back into the floor and draw your lower abdominals up. At the same time, lifting your chest and shoulders off the floor, draw your upper and lower abdominals together. Keep pressing your back firmly into the floor.

Pause, holding your tummy muscles in and squeezing deeply into your abdomen. Slowly, keeping tension in your muscles, lower yourself back to the start position.

Lightly touch the floor with your shoulder blades, then repeat. Work the stated number of repetitions and sets.

ABDOMINAL STRETCH

Breathe normally throughout.

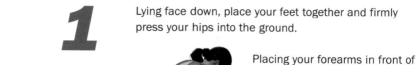

1 Lying face down, place your feet together and firmly press your hips into the ground.

Placing your forearms in front of you, rest them with the palms of your hands flat on the ground.

2 Very slowly lift your chest off the floor, taking care to keep your chin tucked in and your head aligned with your spine. Pull in your stomach muscles.

As you slowly lift the chest, gently pull your torso forward and upward from the ribcage, feeling the tummy stretching. Ensure that your remain firmly pressed to the ground, and that your head is aligned with your spine.

There should be no pressure in your lower back. If there is, you may be moving too far upwards, with your hips lifting off the ground. Think about what you are doing, and where you are meant to be feeling it.

If you want to increase the stretch, bring your arms closer to you.

Hold the stretch for 8 to 10 seconds when you warm up, or for 20 to 30 seconds as part of your cool down, then relax.

Fitness for the day
Walk 25 mins
You have almost reached the maximum number of repetitions on these first five exercises. Well done – this is fantastic!

Exercise 1: Wall press 24–26 reps, 3 sets
Exercise 2: Leg extension 22–24 reps, 3 sets
Exercise 3: Lower abdomen raise 20–22 reps, 3 sets
Exercise 4: Tricep extension 18–20 reps, 3 sets
Exercise 5: Shoulder shrug 16–18 reps, 3 sets

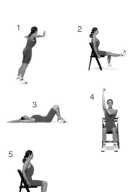

FEELING SCALE FOR EXERCISE

20 MAXIMUM EXERTION

19 EXTRA HARD

17 VERY HARD

16 HARDER

15 HARD

12 LIGHT

10 VERY LIGHT

Food for the day

Breakfast

Snack

Lunch

Snack

Evening meal
Paella. Go easy on the oil, add a few strands of saffron and anything you find in the fridge – chopped cold chicken, prawns, white fish, vegetables, tomatoes and so on

Light snack

★ Goal for the week
You're nearing the end of the 12 weeks – make your goal really hard this week!

★ Fitness goal
How about getting a friend to walk with you?

Mood for the day
Mood at the start of the day
Mood at the end of the day

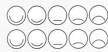

Food tips
Keep the lid on when you are poaching food; this keeps more liquid in the pan and means you need less fat to keep food moist.

Motivation tips
Don't act on the wishes of others – this is all about you.

Fitness for the day
Walk 25-26 mins

Pump your arms to get them up above your heart. You should be feeling more relaxed about using your arms and less worried about how you look doing it by now. Who cares how it looks? Your purpose is to enjoy yourself and reap some benefits for your body. You are nearly through this programme – make the most of it.

★ Food goal
How about changing to a lower - fat milk?

FEELING SCALE FOR EXERCISE

20
MAXIMUM EXERTION

19
EXTRA HARD

17
VERY HARD

16
HARDER

15
HARD

12
LIGHT

10
VERY LIGHT

Food for the day

Breakfast

Snack

Lunch

Snack

Evening meal

Light snack

Hot and spicy salsa dip with chopped fresh fruit and vegetable crudités

★ Goal for the week
How's it going?

Mood for the day

Mood at the start of the day

Mood at the end of the day

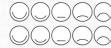

Fitness tips
Pelvic tilts support your torso and improve your sex life – they are definitely worth doing.

Motivation tips
You are nearly there – don't give up now.

WEEK ELEVEN DAY THREE

Fitness for the day
Walk 26 mins

Look back at the photographs of these exercises to be sure that you are not missing anything out. As you do each exercise, think about your posture, which muscles you are working and how you feel them work. Could you slow an exercise down to make it harder? Could you resist more? Think first!

Exercise 1: Wall press 24–26 reps, 3 sets
Exercise 2: Leg extension 22–24 reps, 3 sets
Exercise 3: Lower abdomen raise 20–22 reps, 3 sets
Exercise 4: Tricep extension 18–20 reps, 3 sets
Exercise 5: Shoulder shrug 16–18 reps, 3 sets

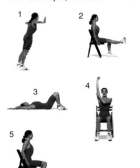

FEELING SCALE FOR EXERCISE

20 MAXIMUM EXERTION

19 EXTRA HARD

17 VERY HARD

16 HARDER

15 HARD

12 LIGHT

10 VERY LIGHT

Food for the day

Breakfast

Snack

Lunch
Pasta with spinach, ricotta and pine kernels

Snack

Evening meal

Light snack

★ Goal for the week
Keep it up!

★ Food goal
Have you tried making a fat-free salad dressing?

Mood for the day
Mood at the start of the day
Mood at the end of the day

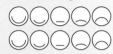

Fitness tips
Think of all the activities you want to try and keep at it; you too can hang glide if you want to.

Motivation tips
Exercise is almost part of your daily life – don't give up now.

140

Fitness for the day
Walk 26-27 mins
Only another 3 minutes to go and then you will have completed your walking goal of 30 minutes. Be sure to focus on using your legs, keep your mind on getting the best workout you can in the time you have. Make those legs do the work, and make those buttocks work for you.

★ Fitness goal
Give yourself a real challenge!

FEELING SCALE FOR EXERCISE

20 MAXIMUM EXERTION

19 EXTRA HARD

17 VERY HARD

16 HARDER

15 HARD

12 LIGHT

10 VERY LIGHT

Food for the day
Breakfast

Snack

Lunch

Snack

Jacket potato – yes, again! They are such a good food

Evening meal

Light snack

★ Goal for the week
Are you on course to achieve your goal?

Mood for the day
Mood at the start of the day

Mood at the end of the day

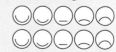

Food tips
Never skip a meal; it won't get rid of excess weight and will make you more likely to head for junk snacks to compensate.

Motivation tips
Never be afraid to join in; try it – you might like it.

Fitness for the day
Walk 27 mins

The new exercise today is excellent for the abdominals, so focus your attention on squeezing deep into your tummy muscles, and taking the emphasis away from your neck. Relax your head into your hands, so that your hands act as a pillow. Don't force or jerk your head forward.

Exercise 6: Calf raise
14–16 reps, 3 sets
Exercise 7: Bicep curl
12–14 reps, 2 sets
Exercise 8: Hamstring curl
10–12 reps, 2 sets
Exercise 9: Shoulder press
8–10 reps, 2 sets
Exercise 10: Chair squat
6–8 reps, 2 sets
Exercise 11: Abdominal curl
4–6 reps, 1 set

FEELING SCALE FOR EXERCISE

20
MAXIMUM EXERTION

19
EXTRA HARD

17
VERY HARD

16
HARDER

15
HARD

12
LIGHT

10
VERY LIGHT

Food for the day

Breakfast

Snack

Lunch
Rice salad – add chopped turkey, raw vegetables, raisins, fresh fruit, seeds, nuts ... the choice is endless

Snack

Evening meal

Light snack

★ Goal for the week
Still feeling good?

★ Food goal
How about trying an exotic vegetable you haven't bought before?

Mood for the day
Mood at the start of the day
Mood at the end of the day
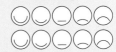

6
7
8

9
10
11

Fitness tips
When you think you can't manage another rep, try one. You may surprise yourself.

Motivation tips
You can if you want to.

Fitness for the day
Walk 27-28 mins

This is great – you are so nearly there! Push hard today and keep your workout up in the 16–17 range on the feeling scale. Get your heart pumping and your body burning fat. Keep an eye on your posture.

★ Fitness goal

To get your partner or your children out walking with you.

FEELING SCALE FOR EXERCISE

20 MAXIMUM EXERTION

19 EXTRA HARD

17 VERY HARD

16 HARDER

15 HARD

12 LIGHT

10 VERY LIGHT

Food for the day

Breakfast

Snack

Cereal bar – check out the health food shops for the best selections

Lunch

Snack

Evening meal

Light snack

★ Goal for the week

Almost there – don't give up.

Mood for the day

Mood at the start of the day

Mood at the end of the day

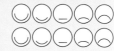

Food tips

Aim for variety: one day take lunch from home, the next use the canteen (but watch what you eat), the next make a delicious sandwich and so on.

Motivation tips

Familiarity makes you bored. Try something new.

Fitness for the day
Walk 28-30 mins

Into the third sets of both calf raises and biceps curls – you must be feeling good. Keep it up. Today is also the day that you hit that golden 30 minutes, prepared for week 12.

Exercise 6: Calf raise
14–16 reps, 3 sets
Exercise 7: Bicep curl
12–14 reps, 2 sets
Exercise 8: Hamstring curl
10–12 reps, 2 sets
Exercise 9: Shoulder press
reps 8–10, sets 2
Exercise 10: Chair squat
6–8 reps, 2 sets
Exercise 11: Abdominal curl
4–6 reps 1, sets

FEELING SCALE FOR EXERCISE

20
MAXIMUM EXERTION

19
EXTRA HARD

17
VERY HARD

16
HARDER

15
HARD

12
LIGHT

10
VERY LIGHT

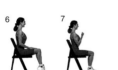

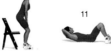

Food for the day

Breakfast

Snack

Lunch

Snack

Evening meal

Couscous with vegetable and bean casserole; if you buy pre-cooked couscous it only needs steaming to be ready – and even the kids will love it

Light snack

★ Goal for the week
Well, did you manage it?

★ Food goal
Are you still drinking alcohol more than a couple of times a week?

Mood for the day

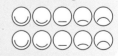

Mood at the start of the day

Mood at the end of the day

Fitness tips
Count down when the reps get high – it's very difficult to stop at six when you know you should go five, four, three, two, one.

Motivation tips
Learn to like yourself – you have every reason to do so.

WEEK TWELVE INTRODUCTION

This is it – the final week, hip hip hooray! This programme has brought you from doing nothing to achieving a good 30-minute walk daily, which I am sure has not been plain sailing. Congratulate yourself on making the effort and realizing your potential. Look back over the diary for the first week, when you walked only 2 minutes – can you believe you have come this far? Well believe it and believe that you can now, if you put your mind to it, and your heart into it, do what ever you want to. You have chosen and realized sensible goals and appreciated what that can do for you.

This week you are firmly anchoring that 30-minute walk into your daily schedule, which is necessary if you want to maintain this level of fitness. Work hard over the week to walk as well as you can, making every stride count. Remember that your arms are an integral part of walking. The moment you drop them below the level of your heart, your heart rate falls too, which means that you are not working at a high intensity – perhaps only as high as 13–14 on the feeling scale. Go out and enjoy the sensation of walking at a brisk pace, without feeling breathless and uncomfortable.

At the end of this week, you have your final assessment (pp. 155–6) which will show you how you have progressed in your quest to reduce your body fat. From the assessment you will be able to see how you have been affected by your moods and how these have been influenced by the number of walks and the amount of exercises you have done. Has changing your eating habits shown you how much you are influenced by food? Have your moods changed? How are your goals? Have you reached your first set, or are you still working hard at them? Time is on your side, so don't worry about how long it takes to reach them: the important thing is that you do. When you fill in the end-of-month assessment, you will see for yourself how your food goals and eating habits have changed for the better over the 12 weeks. You now have to decide what to do next too, so think about that as you work through the week.

Your last exercise is the lower back raise. The muscles in this area do not show the effect of exercise in the same way as those of your arms or legs, but this exercise still has an important part to play. The lower-back muscles support the front and back of your body. Excess weight around your abdomen puts pressure on your back, which can lead to injury, especially if your lower back is weak. So get to it!

LOWER BACK RAISE

1 This is a very subtle exercise, so treat it with respect. Check your posture throughout and remember that the movement you are making should be small.

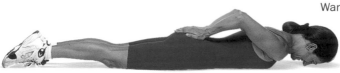

Warm up and stretch.

Lie face down, with your feet together and hips pressed firmly into the floor.

Pull your tummy in and place your hands on your buttocks. Tighten your buttocks and hold this position.

Tuck your chin toward your chest so that your head is in line with your spine and not straining to look upward.

2 Breathe in and out, then breathe in again. This time, as you breathe out, slowly and gently raise your chest off the floor. Use the muscles of your lower back to lift.

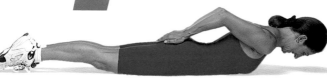

Pause. Keep your hips on the floor and don't jerk upward – the movement should be small and you should not feel any discomfort in your lower back. If you do, you are lifting too high so stop, lower back to the start position and start again.

Work the stated number of repetitions and sets.

LOWER BACK STRETCH

1

This is a lovely relaxing stretch, one to do often, especially if you sit or stand in the same position all day.

Breathe normally throughout.

Sitting on the floor, bend both knees and place your feet flat on the floor, hip width apart. Slide your feet forward slightly.

Keep your head aligned with your spine and your shoulders relaxed.

2

Slowly bend the upper body forward, curving your back. Place both your hands behind your knees or on your ankles, and bring your knees towards your chest.

Hold this position and feel the tension in your lower back and buttocks easing away. Relax your neck and shoulders.

Hold the stretch for 8 to 10 seconds when you warm up, and for 20 to 30 seconds as part of the cool down, then relax.

WEEK TWELVE DAY ONE

Fitness for the day
Walk 30 mins

You have now reached the maximum number of repetitions this week, of the wall press – haven't you come a long way? Continue to focus on the muscles you are working. Take your time and do each exercise slowly, resisting the movements up and down on all reps and all sets.

Exercise 1: Wall press
26–30 reps, 3 sets
Exercise 2: Leg extension
24–26 reps, 3 sets
Exercise 3: Lower abdomen
raise 22–24 reps, 3 sets
Exercise 4: Tricep extension
20–22 reps, 3 sets
Exercise 5: Shoulder shrug
18–20 reps, 3 sets
Exercise 6: Calf raise
16–18 reps, 3 sets

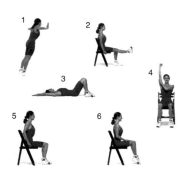

FEELING SCALE FOR EXERCISE

20 MAXIMUM EXERTION

19 EXTRA HARD

17 VERY HARD

16 HARDER

15 HARD

12 LIGHT

10 VERY LIGHT

Food for the day

Breakfast

Snack

Lunch
Stir-fry vegetables with tofu

Snack

Evening meal

Light snack

★ Goal for the week
This is it – the final week – your last chance to prove you CAN do it!

★ Fitness goal
To try one new leisure activity.

Mood for the day

Mood at the start of the day
Mood at the end of the day

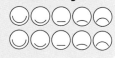

Food tips
Aim for at least five portions of fruit and vegetables every day – juicing some of them makes sense.

Motivation tips
Keep busy, keep moving, keep fit.

148

Fitness for the day
Walk 30 mins

Believe in yourself, you have the willpower, which comes from within. Use this 30 minutes as maintenance for your body and for your mind. Continue to keep in the 15--16-17 range on the feeling scale – the harder you work, the more effective you will be. Enjoy the high that this 30-minute walk gives you.

★ Food goal

How about checking out the local health-food shop? You may find something you like?

FEELING SCALE FOR EXERCISE

20 MAXIMUM EXERTION

19 EXTRA HARD

17 VERY HARD

16 HARDER

15 HARD

12 LIGHT

10 VERY LIGHT

Food for the day

Breakfast

Snack

Lunch

Snack

Fresh fruit salad – as much as you can eat

Evening meal

Light snack

★ Goal for the week

Really go for it this week – you know you can do it!

Mood for the day

Mood at the start of the day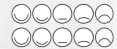

Mood at the end of the day

Fitness tips

Keep your running shoes in the car / at the office. You may be inspired to go for a run.

Motivation tips

Each step does make a difference.

Fitness for the day
Walk 30 mins

You should be feeling and seeing the results of your hard work on these exercises over the last 12 weeks. You have probably found some easier than others and you almost certainly have some favourites (you have favourites – now there's a good sign!). Focus your attention on the ones you find more difficult, and eventually – as your muscles slowly get stronger and you are better able to cope – they will cease to be so difficult.

Exercise 1: Wall press 26–30 reps, 3 sets
Exercise 2: Leg extension 24–26 reps, 3 sets
Exercise 3: Lower abdomen raise 22–24 reps, sets 3
Exercise 4: Tricep extension 20–22 reps, 3 sets
Exercise 5: Shoulder shrug 18–20 reps, 3 sets
Exercise 6: Calf raise 16–18 reps, 3 sets

FEELING SCALE FOR EXERCISE
20 MAXIMUM EXERTION
19 EXTRA HARD
17 VERY HARD
16 HARDER
15 HARD
12 LIGHT
10 VERY LIGHT

Food for the day

Breakfast

Snack
Wholemeal currant and raisin scones

Lunch

Snack

Evening meal

Light snack

★ **Goal for the week**
Still on target?

★ **Food goal**
Try a different sort of mineral water – there are dozens to choose from.

Mood for the day

Mood at the start of the day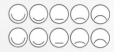
Mood at the end of the day

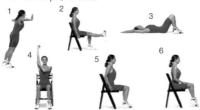

Fitness tips
Your body is like the car engine – sometimes it needs pampering.

Motivation tips
Boredom triggers bad habits; if you feel bored, go for a walk, run a bath – anything to head off a bad habit.

Fitness for the day
Walk 30 mins

You have reached your first major goal, that of improving your all-round physical and emotional fitness. But it is important to continue to challenge your body when you walk and to carry on using this time as time on your own, just for you. Good posture should be automatic, but don't stop checking yourself – it's surprising how quickly you can slide back into old habits.

★ Fitness goal

Do you do your walk if it's raining or put it off? Try it, you may like it.

FEELING SCALE FOR EXERCISE

20
MAXIMUM EXERTION

19
EXTRA HARD

17
VERY HARD

16
HARDER

15
HARD

12
LIGHT

10
VERY LIGHT

Food for the day

Breakfast

Snack

Lunch

Snack

Evening meal

Mixed bean casserole; use everything you put in a meat version except beef stock (use vegetable) and meat (use beans – any or all you like)

Light snack

★ Goal for the week

Are you on course to achieve it?

Mood for the day

Mood at the start of the day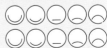

Mood at the end of the day

Food tips

If you find it difficult to give up butter, try moistening bread with tomato purée, horseradish or mustard.

Motivation tips

Live for the present and the future, not the past.

Fitness for the day
Walk 30 mins

Up to three sets of hamstring curls – congratulations! Work hard at all the exercises, keep reminding yourself how you have worked hard to increase the repetitions and sets, to get this far. This week's new exercise, the lower back raise, complements last week's abdominal curl. Strengthening this area will help to keep your torso upright and help alleviate backache.

Exercise 7: Bicep curl
14–16 reps, 3 sets
Exercise 8: Hamstring curl
12–14 reps, 3 sets
Exercise 9: Shoulder press
10–12 reps, 2 sets
Exercise 10: Chair squat
8–10 reps, 2 sets
Exercise 11: Abdominal curl
6–8 reps, 2 sets
Exercise 12: Lower back raise
4–6 reps, 1 set

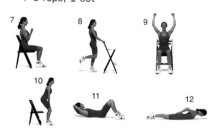

FEELING SCALE FOR EXERCISE

20 MAXIMUM EXERTION

19 EXTRA HARD

17 VERY HARD

16 HARDER

15 HARD

12 LIGHT

10 VERY LIGHT

Food for the day

Breakfast
Porridge with soya milk and apple juice

Snack

Lunch

Snack

Evening meal

Light snack

★ Goal for the week
Almost there – don't give up!

★ Food goal
Have you bought your non-stick frying pan?

Mood for the day
Mood at the start of the day
Mood at the end of the day
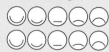

Fitness tips
When you find the going tough, visualize your muscles as you want them to be.

Motivation tips
Life is too short for regrets – get on and do it now.

Fitness for the day
Walk 30 mins

This is such an achievement – you must praise yourself for coming so far. This 30 minutes daily walk will help you to think more clearly and feel greater control over your actions. Bask in the knowledge that you are burning fuel, energizing your system, burning fat and feeling good for it. Stride out for a better life.

★ Fitness goal

To play with the children in the park – not just watch while they play.

FEELING SCALE FOR EXERCISE

20
MAXIMUM EXERTION

19
EXTRA HARD

17
VERY HARD

16
HARDER

15
HARD

12
LIGHT

10
VERY LIGHT

Food for the day

Breakfast

Snack

Lunch

Snack

Evening meal

Spicy potato bake – add onions, nutmeg, yogurt and any other vegetables you like

Light snack

★ Goal for the week

Keep it up – you're doing brilliantly!

Mood for the day

Mood at the start of the day

Mood at the end of the day

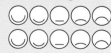

Food tips
Don't slide back into bad habits. Why waste all your efforts?

Motivation tips
You can do anything you want – haven't you proved it already?

Fitness for the day
Walk 30 mins

Take the lower back raises gently. You may not feel as if they are doing anything for you, but take your time and do them well – your lower back needs to be looked after. Respect your body and it will do anything for you. And, again, congratulations – you have done absolutely brilliantly!

Exercise 7: Bicep curl
14–16 reps, 3 sets
Exercise 8: Hamstring curl
12–14 reps, 3 sets
Exercise 9: Shoulder press
10–12 reps, 2 sets
Exercise 10: Chair squat
8–10 reps 2 sets
Exercise 11: Abdominal curl
6–8 reps, 2 sets
Exercise 12: Lower back raise
4–6 reps, 2 sets

FEELING SCALE FOR EXERCISE

20 MAXIMUM EXERTION

19 EXTRA HARD

17 VERY HARD

16 HARDER

15 HARD

12 LIGHT

10 VERY LIGHT

Food for the day
Breakfast

Snack

Lunch
Tuna pasta bake; make a crispy topping from a small amount of cheese and grated brown breadcrumbs

Snack

Evening meal

Light snack

★ Goal for the week
Have you made it? Fantastic – what an achievement!

★ Food goal
To treat my tastebuds.

Mood for the day

Mood at the start of the day

Mood at the end of the day

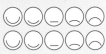

Fitness tips
Don't worry about the next set. Concentrate on the one you are doing.

Motivation tips
You don't need one – you are a star!

It's that time again, with the difference that you have now completed the whole twelve-week programme and must know by now what some of your results are going to show. You feel better, don't you? And you know that you look better. However, fill in the assessment so that you have a complete record of the programme. Look back on them in six months time, when you are even closer to some of your long-term goals and remind yourself how far you have come.

Fitness and food assessment

At the end of each week add up how many times you reached your goal and note it on the grid. Do your results show a steady improvement over the twelve weeks, or did it go in fits and starts? You may have noticed that you

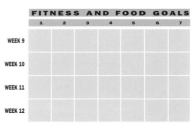

FITNESS AND FOOD GOALS

	1	2	3	4	5	6	7
WEEK 9							
WEEK 10							
WEEK 11							
WEEK 12							

reached fewer goals when you increased the pace of your workouts, or increased the length of your walk, or tried to tackle a really stubborn food habit. Don't be disheartened – this is natural.

6–7 goals per week
Excellent – you will not give up after all this hard work, will you? What are you going to do next? Join a gym, try a little circuit training perhaps, or some cross training? Or buy a fitness video. The choice is yours, but whatever you do, bring the same dedication you have shown over these weeks to it. Remind yourself how good you feel today if you are tempted to fall back into old habits.

4–5 goals per week
Very good. Keep at it and you will find that as you lay more habits to rest, your success rate in your goals snowballs. Move on to something different, or repeat the last couple of weeks exercises for the next month to really consolidate what you have built up so far.

3 goals per week
Good. Is this an improvement on last month, or about the same? If you seem stuck make your goals a bit easier – you need the boost of getting there more often.

1–2 goals per week
Keep trying, but be prepared for changes to take a while longer. Well done for sticking with it, you have proved you have willpower.

ASSESSMENT

Feeling scale assessment

Add up the entries on your feeling scales and note them on the grid. If you are slipping below 15, increase your resistance as you exercise and pump your arms harder as you walk, to increase the effort you make.

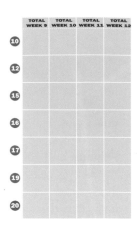

Mood scale assessment

Fill in the mood grids for the beginning and end of each day. Are your moods improving overall? Look back to see how you scored at the end of month two and month one. What a difference! You know good food, exercise and a healthy lifestyle improve your sense of well being – keep at it.

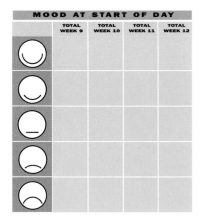

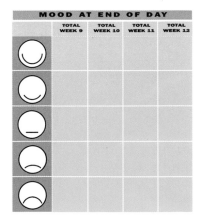

INDEX

INDEX

O

oxygen 13, 14, 17, 26, 30, 31

P

pain 27
pasta 20, 29
pelvic floor muscles 28
pelvis 8, 28
posture 8, 16, 28, 51, 125
    in the car 9
    movement 8
    rest 8
    at work 9
potatoes 20
protein 21
    sources of
        dairy products 21
        eggs 21
        white meats 21
pulse monitor 13

Q

quadriceps 103
quick weight loss 5

R

retirement 14
rice 21, 29

S

salad 20
shoes 17
shoulders 10
shoulder press
    see exercises
shoulder shrug
    see exercises
smoking
    see cigarettes
snacks 20
sportswear 17-18
stomach 51
strength training 10

stress incontinence 28
stretches
    abdominal 137
    bicep 95
    buttocks 127
    calf 85
    chest 33
    front of thigh 43
    hamstring 105
    lower abdominal raise 53
    lower back 147
    tricep 63
stretching 17
sugar 25
synovial fluids 16

T

tea 24
thighs 11, 41
toe taps 83
tricep extension
    see exercises
tricep stretch 63

U

upper body 10
    see bicep curl,
        shoulder press,
        shoulder shrug, tricep
        extension, wall press

V

vegetables 20, 29

W

wall press
    see exercises
warm up 13, 16-17
white meats 21
wholemeal bread 21, 29